MOSBY'S DENTAL PRACTICE MANAGEMENT SERIES

Personalized guide to practice evaluation

MOSBY'S DENTAL PRACTICE MANAGEMENT SERIES

Personalized guide to practice evaluation

Editors

THOMAS L. SNYDER, D.M.D., M.B.A.
President

CHARLES J. FELMEISTER, D.M.D., M.B.A.
Executive Vice President

Snyder Felmeister and Co.
Cherry Hill, New Jersey

Authors

Thomas L. Snyder, D.M.D., M.B.A.

Larry R. Domer, D.B.A., M.B.A.

Associate Professor, Department of Applied Dentistry,
University of Colorado, School of Dentistry,
Denver, Colorado

The C. V. Mosby Company

ST. LOUIS • TORONTO • LONDON   1983

MOSBY

A TRADITION OF PUBLISHING EXCELLENCE

Editor: Darlene Warfel
Assistant editor: Melba Steube
Editing supervisor: Lin Dempsey Hallgren
Manuscript editor: Diane Ackermann
Book design: Kay M. Kramer
Cover design: Diane Beasley
Production: Carol O'Leary, Susan Trail

Printed in the United States of America

The C.V. Mosby Company
11830 Westline Industrial Drive, St. Louis, Missouri 63141

Library of Congress Cataloging in Publication Data

Snyder, Thomas L.
    Personalized guide to practice evaluation.

    (Mosby's dental practice management series; v. 1)
    Includes index.
    1. Dentistry—Practice. I. Felmeister, Charles J.
II. Domer, Larry R. III. Title. IV. Series.
[DNLM: 1. Practice management, Dental. WU 77 S675p]
RK58.S58   1983   617.6′0068   82-14306
ISBN 0-8016-4715-0

AC/VH/VH 9 8 7 6 5 4 3 2 1   02/D/217

Preface

Today's economy and the changing dental marketplace have resulted in an increasing emphasis on the importance of dental practice management. The difficulty of maintaining your standard of living, the increasing supply of dental personpower, and the competition brought about by new dental delivery methods are but a few realities confronting you, the dental practitioner.

The past years of double-digit inflation, continually high interest rates, and the apparent declining business in many dental practices make it increasingly difficult to properly manage your practice and to derive from it the satisfaction that dentistry as a career was to provide you.

For the recent graduate, establishing your own private practice has been more complex and risk laden. Locating a suitable location, especially in metropolitan areas for general practitioners and specialists alike is very difficult indeed. Obtaining the appropriate level of financial support from commercial lending institutions and private financing companies is not as routine and as relatively easy a task that it was in years past. In fact many lenders look very critically at your financial status, often demanding a well designed bank plan that includes a rationale for your practice location decision.

Although this scenario has caused some dentists to conclude that the "golden years of dentistry" are over and that the profession's future is bleak, we, as authors of this series, do not agree. Dental practices *can* and *will* survive and thrive in the future! For this to happen, you must become more proficient and knowledgeable in the management and marketing of your practice. Our opinion is based on a significant number of practices that are presently experiencing positive growth and achieving high levels of financial success. In most instances, these practices are owned by dentists who have developed expertise in managing their practices, who understand and have developed effective marketing strategies, who use competent professional resources, and who are willing to experiment and make changes in their practices.

The development of management expertise is, however, not achieved quickly. It requires a considerable investment in time and effort and an insatiable appetite to read and learn about dental practice management. Meeting these requirements is difficult for most practicing dentists and is even more difficult for senior dental students and recent dental graduates. Although no one but you can control the time and effort you devote to developing management expertise, this workbook and the others in this series should serve as an excellent primer to focus on specific problems that you now face or that you will face in the near future and provide a framework for sound practice management decision making.

Thomas L. Snyder
Larry R. Domer

Contents

MOSBY'S DENTAL PRACTICE MANAGEMENT SERIES

Personalized guide to practice evaluation

Introduction

PURPOSE OF WORKBOOK

This workbook provides information concerning the various practice management systems that will be of value to established practitioners as well as new dentists. The diagnostic surveys and the self-scoring system used in Part I enables established practitioners to analyze their present level of management sophistication and offers concrete suggestions for improvement. Part II of the text provides information and worksheets that will help new dentists to evaluate practice alternatives and make sound decisions in developing and establishing a new practice. This portion of the workbook can also assist dentists who want to establish additional or multiple practice locations.

The emphasis in this workbook is on decision making and problem identification. Thus minimal attention is paid to detailed philosophical and theoretical presentations. Information of this nature is provided in *Dental Practice Management: Concepts and Applications,* by Larry R. Domer, Thomas L. Snyder, and David W. Heid (St. Louis, 1980, The C.V. Mosby Co.). Decision making and problem identification have been combined in this workbook because they are the two most important prerequisites for developing and maintaining an economically successful dental practice. Starting your practice without making major errors in judgment is of paramount importance to developing a successful practice. After your practice is established, one of the most important components in managing it successfully is by conducting ongoing evaluations and analyses. These analyses provide the basis for identifying problems and opportunities and for making those changes that are necessary to ensure the continued growth and efficiency of your practice. Intelligent decisions concerning changes in patient care, finances, personnel, or marketing are not possible unless you can systematically evaluate your practice's past and present performance and compare it with the goals and objectives that you have established.

WORKBOOK DESIGN

Because the major purposes of this workbook are to assist you in analyzing your practice or to facilitate your starting a practice, it primarily consists of tools designed to accomplish these ends. These tools are in the form of worksheets, checklists, and charts, and each has been designed with a specific purpose in mind. In most cases, this purpose is to provide a framework for analyzing a particular problem and making a logical decision concerning its resolution. In other instances, the worksheets allow you to rate and compare yourself with minimum levels of management performance that are necessary for practice success. These tools should facilitate the identification of issues related to various problems and decisions you will encounter in managing your practice or in starting a new practice.

Finally, whether you are completing Part 1 or Part II of this workbook, allocate enough time so that you can complete at least one chapter thoroughly in each working session. The directions are written clearly and the worksheets are designed so that you can minimize time, yet obtain the results you need to improve your proficiency in practice management and planning.

Part one
Analysis of an existing dental practice

Any dental practice occasionally encounters managerial and operational problems. A key to resolving them is to use an organized method to assess all major practice management areas within your practice and to determine the degree to which each may require some improvement.

Part I of this workbook, "Analysis of an existing dental practice," provides a systematic approach for you and your staff to assess your practice's policies and procedures and the degree to which they are implemented (Fig. 1). This assessment is accomplished by the completion of worksheets for each practice management area. If you score below a predetermined score, you can refer to Chapter 10, which provides recommendations for improvement in each area. The practice management areas that you will be analyzing are:

Collection procedures
Appointment scheduling
Recall program analysis
Personnel management
Inventory system analysis
Laboratory flow analysis
Bookkeeping/accounting system analysis
Practice building
Financial management

Each of these areas consists of key factors that are essential to effective practice management in any office. Although all practices will not utilize each factor to the same degree, successful practices utilize each to an acceptable level of performance. As you complete the worksheets, you may discover that many factors we have identified are not being utilized to the degree we believe they should. If you score below our acceptable standard, you can refer to Chapter 10, which provides you with some recommendations we think can assist you in improving a practice management area. To develop the worksheets, we have utilized a practice analysis model as seen in Fig. 2 to help you identify your practice's strengths and weakness and to pinpoint recommendations for identified problems concerning important factors.

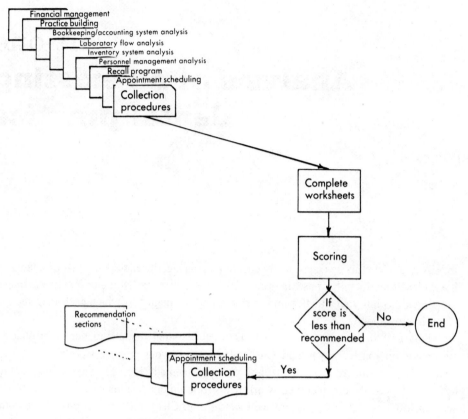

Fig. 1. Practice analysis protocol.

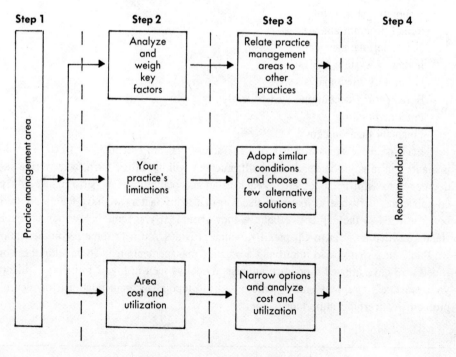

Fig. 2. Practice analysis model.

To use the workbook, instead of starting with the first chapter and proceeding in sequence to the last, we suggest that you complete the worksheet below, then turn to the chapter that you rated 9 and complete the worksheets. Continue through your priority list until you complete the entire practice analysis.

MANAGEMENT AREA PRIORITIES

Directions: Rate each practice management area listed below according to its importance in your practice. Select the most important (9), next important (8), and so on by using the following scale:

9 = Most important
1 = Least important

	Importance	Page No.
Collection procedures	_____	6
Appointment scheduling	_____	13
Recall program analysis	_____	19
Personnel management	_____	22
Inventory system analysis	_____	29
Laboratory flow analysis	_____	33
Bookkeeping/accounting system analysis	_____	37
Practice building	_____	42
Financial management	_____	48

COMPLETING THE WORKSHEETS

The worksheets are designed to be easily scored. The scoring mechanism will allow you to compare the various systems in your practice to a model practice, which was developed through extensive experience with a wide range of dental practices. When completing each worksheet:

1. Answer each question as accurately as possible.
2. Use staff input when necessary.

After answering each question in a worksheet section, grade it by multiplying the predetermined question weight by the point value of your response. Total all points for your worksheet score. If your score is less than our recommended score, consult Chapter 10 to review the recommendations for improving that particular practice management area. If these recommendations are insufficient, consider soliciting suggestions from your staff or confer with a management consultant.

1 Collection procedures

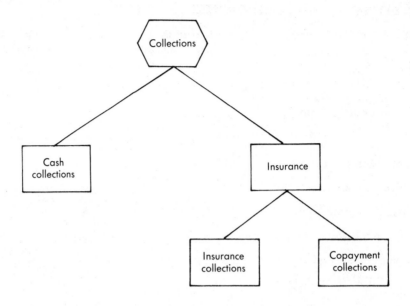

Have you ever experienced not having enough money in your practice's checking account to meet all of your monthly expenses, or were you ever unable to pay yourself the salary or draw for which you had previously planned? These two situations are usually not attributed to low practice productivity but rather to poor cash flow. Collecting payments is often a major problem in dental practices. Whether 70% of your patients are covered by a third party plan or whether the majority of your patients pay for your services ''out of pocket,'' the collection policies and procedures that you established have a critical impact on your cash flow. Also, your patient's perceptions of your overall business skills are established by the manner in which you have organized your collection procedures and the effectiveness which you collect outstanding balances and process insurance claim forms. Because the overwhelming majority of dental practices are affected by dental insurance, any collection procedure must address three major areas: cash collections, insurance collections, and copayment management (see diagram above).

CASH COLLECTIONS

Most accountants and management consultants advise that fees not covered by a third party plan should be collected at the time of treatment. To have an effective policy in this area, your staff must be properly trained to tactfully collect the fee from the patient at the time of treatment. If the fee cannot be collected at the time of treatment, two choices remain: billing for services or payment arrangements. If bills are to be sent, an entire billing system must be established to include at least the type of statement, the frequency of billing, the aging procedure for outstanding balances, and the account follow-up policies and procedures. Payment arrangements may include the calculation of a fixed monthly amount to be paid over a predetermined period. These arrangements are frequently used in high fee situations such as orthodontics and complex periodontal therapy.

Statistical information is also required to properly monitor the effectiveness of your cash collection procedures. Your best monitoring tool is to use an accounts receivable aging report that categorizes the amounts owed over a period of time starting at the day that a particular service is rendered. Usually these account balances are categorized as follows:

   0 to 30 days
   31 to 60 days
   61 to 90 days
   91 to 120 days
   Over 120 days

Knowing the age of each account as well as the overall totals of the practice's outstanding accounts receivable is extremely useful in monitoring the effectiveness of your existing collection policies and procedures.

INSURANCE COLLECTIONS AND COPAYMENT MANAGEMENT

Most urban practices are heavily dependent on dental insurance. Therefore an effective system that permits timely claims processing and submission, in addition to an effective claims follow-up procedure will assure that your practice maintains an even cash flow. Also, a well-organized system for categorizing benefit plans will assist you in maintaining patient rapport by minimizing misunderstandings that frequently occur because of insufficient information regarding your patient's insurance coverage. The major components of insurance collections are depicted in Fig. 3.

The most important aspect of doing business with patients who have dental insurance is to know which deductibles, copayments, annual limitations, and exclusions may exist before you begin treatment or discuss fees for the case. If any of these factors apply to your patient's coverage, arrangements must be made for the collection of any out-of-pocket expenses for the treatment. It is critical that your patient understand his or her financial responsibility before the treatment is begun. Equally important is the submission of any preauthorization forms for cases exceeding a prescribed dollar amount. The appropriate follow-up of any preauthorization is important, especially in cases that may cause disputes with the insurance carrier over treatment recommendations, because such preauthorization may increase your patient's out-of-pocket cost. After determining the level of benefits and any out-of-pocket expenditures, the timely submission of claims becomes the next major factor. This includes the processing of any applicable copayment and the assignment of benefits to the dentist. If you accept assignment on a routine basis, the timely and accurate completion and submission of claim forms is crucial. A follow-up system to monitor pending claims is required to ensure against unnecessary delays in receiving payment from an insurance carrier. Also, a copayment follow-up system is needed for those patients who do not have complete insurance coverage. The steps in this process are depicted in Fig. 4.

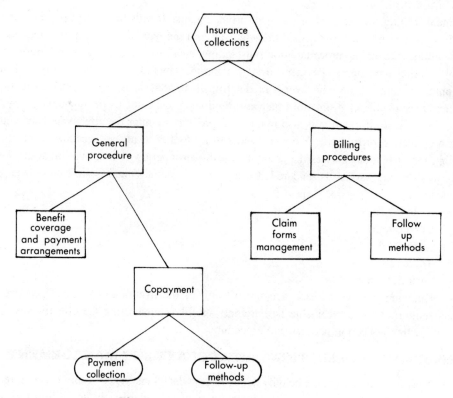

Fig. 3. Insurance collection procedures.

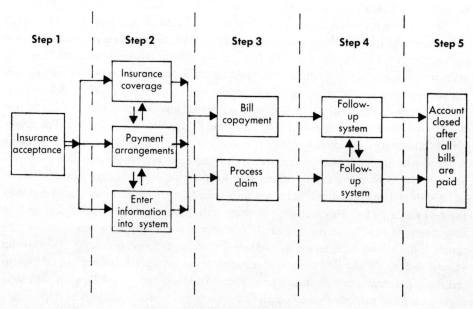

Fig. 4. Insurance processing cycle.

Many patient relation problems are caused by misunderstandings about the patient's out-of-pocket responsibility for services covered in a dental benefit plan. To avoid this, a clear understanding must be established at the first visit before beginning any treatment. You have two choices for handling copayments. The most preferred method is to consider copayments the same as cash collections, using the same procedures outlined earlier in this chapter. The alternative method is to bill the patient for the copayment portion after you have received the claim check from the carrier. One problem with this alternative is the danger that your patient may resent paying for a portion of a service originally thought to be covered totally by the dental benefit plan. This resentment may be caused by the patient forgetting that there was a copayment for a procedure rather than a reluctance to pay you for your service.

In summary, effective insurance collection policies and procedures require careful attention to detail, an efficient system for completing and submitting claims, and an excellent follow-up system to monitor outstanding claims and copayments.

• • •

To assess the effectiveness of your collection procedures, please answer all questions on the collection procedures worksheet. If you cannot answer all the questions yourself, ask your staff to assist you. If you score less than 199, refer to the collection procedures recommendations on p. 55.

COLLECTION PROCEDURES WORKSHEET

Directions: Answer each question by circling the appropriate response. Multiply the weight (W) for each question in the left column by the value of your response: Yes = 2, No = 0. Add the totals in the right-hand column to determine your score (S) for this section.

                                                                   W   **S**

1. Have cash collection procedures been explained to the responsible individual(s) on your staff?   2 Yes   0 No   X   **8** =

2. Are your cash collection procedures in writing?   2 Yes   0 No   X   **4** =

3. Are payment arrangements specified prior to beginning treatment?   2 Yes   0 No   X   **7** =

4. Are payment arrangements specified in writing to your patients?   2 Yes   0 No   X   **4** =

5. Is payment requested at the time of treatment?   2 Yes   0 No   X   **4** =

6. Do you have a follow-up system for late payments?   2 Yes   0 No   X   **5** =

7. Are bills sent to patients at least monthly?   2 Yes   0 No   X   **6** =

8. Do you use a follow-up list for delinquent accounts?   2 Yes   0 No   X   **4** =

COLLECTION PROCEDURES WORKSHEET—cont'd

W   S

9. Do you review your delinquent accounts list at least monthly?   2 Yes 0 No X **7** =

10. Do you take any action such as telephone follow-up or letter writing for your accounts that are overdue past 60 days?   2 Yes 0 No X **5** =

11. Does your staff know the benefits provided for your patients by each carrier?   2 Yes 0 No X **3** =

12. Does your staff know what limitations in coverage a patient may have during the period of 1 year?   2 Yes 0 No X **5** =

13. Do you submit insurance claims at least on a weekly basis?   2 Yes 0 No X **7** =

14. Do you use an insurance follow-up log?   2 Yes 0 No X **5** =

15. Do you or your staff review your insurance log at least monthly?   2 Yes 0 No X **7** =

16. If payment has not been received from the insurance carrier within the normal payment cycle, do you contact the carrier?   2 Yes 0 No X **7** =

17. Do you wait for authorization before beginning major cases?   2 Yes 0 No X **5** =

COLLECTION PROCEDURES WORKSHEET—cont'd

		W	S

18. Is the amount of insurance coverage available discussed with each patient before treatment?

2 Yes
0 No   X   4 =

19. Is the patient informed of any copayment responsibility before treatment?

2 Yes
0 No   X   6 =

20. Do you make specific copayment arrangements before beginning treatment?

2 Yes
0 No   X   5 =

21. When assignment is accepted, do you request copayment during the course of treatment?

2 Yes
0 No   X   6 =

Total _____

2 Appointment scheduling

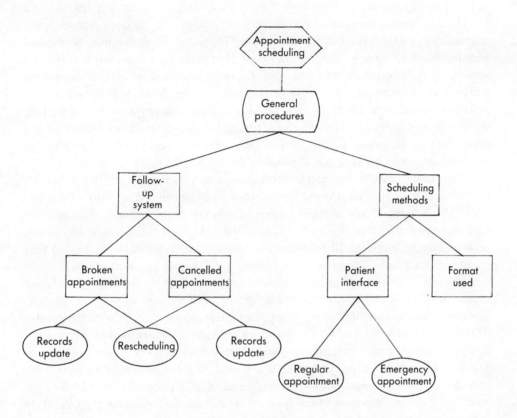

Appointment scheduling and its control form a system that enables the effective coordination of all activities of the dental practice. Although there cannot be an ideal appointment system because of variations in practice size, the type of services provided, and the personal philosophy and work habits of the service providers, the basic concepts of appointment scheduling and control should be present in each system. Appointment scheduling and control consist of two major factors: the method used and the follow-up system. These factors are directly dependent on the policies established, the personnel responsible for scheduling and follow-up, your written records, and physical space limitations.

The goals of any appointment scheduling system should include (1) controlling the flow of patients, (2) minimizing the dentist's slack time, (3) utilizing auxiliary personnel efficiently, (4) providing a full but unrushed schedule, and (5) keeping the dentist and the patients on time.

Appointment scheduling for each patient may appear to be a relatively simple procedure; however, it is actually quite complex. Patient appointment scheduling requires many decisions to be made from a number of alternatives. The receptionist requires carefully developed written policies as a guide for making the best decision. Appointment scheduling decisions are usually made very quickly yet must take into account considerable information such as the patient's personality, the patient's preference for time and day, and the type of care to be provided. The patient's demands must be matched with the practice's policies, which must consider (1) the time required to perform a service, (2) the practice's work load capacity, (3) the limitations by time of day for the performance of certain procedures, (4) the available operating hours, and (5) the treatment procedures already scheduled for a particular day. Although the physical act of scheduling an appointment appears to be simple, the contingencies and limitations placed on that appointment by the patient and the practice make it difficult. An overview of an effective appointment scheduling system is depicted in the diagram on p. 13.

The methods used for appointment scheduling may vary for each practice. However, regardless of your practice size and type, certain fundamental policies should be developed. All treatments should be planned in such a way that time estimates can be made for each set of procedures that you wish to have scheduled for a particular visit. This is best accomplished by analyzing all procedures in your practice in terms of the average time requirements needed to complete each of them. You can then decide the most common denominator (5 minutes, 10 minutes, 15 minutes) for performing the tasks of each procedure, which will enable you to schedule appointments by units of time. In addition, you must consider whether to schedule appointments by operatory or by doctor/hygienist. This decision is dependent on the physical design and equipment status of each operatory. The third consideration is the design of the appointment book: (1) the number of columns that are required, (2) if procedure codes are used on the appointment sheet, (3) the variation of practice hours (day vs evening), and (4) if a color code is used for each provider. It is also important to consider the mechanism for communicating the daily schedule to the staff and the doctor and the procedure for communicating last minute changes. Of equal importance is the transmittal of information regarding the requirements for future appointments between the receptionist and the doctor.

A major problem in many practices is the handling of emergency patients. This can disrupt what is thought to be a well-planned schedule. It can also infuriate your regularly scheduled patients. It is critical to establish a policy that identifies and defines a true dental emergency and sets guidelines for scheduling such a patient. A weekly analysis of the frequency of emergencies and their impact on the daily schedule will help to plan which time of day is best to allocate time for emergencies.

Equally important to the physical act of scheduling appointments are the follow-up systems that are needed to ensure that maximum productivity can be achieved. The practice's ability to handle broken appointments is extremely critical since this is the least controllable aspect of appointment scheduling. Appropriate policies for handling patients who frequently break appointments must be developed. Your appointment scheduling procedures should also include steps for refilling broken appointments on a last minute basis. Therefore lists of patients who can be on call with short notice can be extremely valuable in practices with a significant problem of broken appointments. Although cancelled appointments can adversely affect the appointment schedule, usually there is lead time available to fill an appointment in that time slot. It is therefore critical to have clearly defined policies and standardized procedures for handling any contingency regarding scheduling for regular patients as well as for new, recall, or emergency patients.

• • •

To assess the effectiveness of your appointment scheduling and control system, please answer all questions on the appointment scheduling worksheet. If you cannot answer all the questions yourself, ask your receptionist to assist you. If you score less than 141, refer to the appointment scheduling recommendations on p. 57.

APPOINTMENT SCHEDULING WORKSHEET

Directions:
1. Answer each question by circling the appropriate response. Multiply the weight (W) for each question in the left column by the value of your response, Yes = 2, No = 0. Add the totals in the right-hand column to determine your score (S) for this section.
2. Important definitions. To respond properly to the questions in this section, please use the following definitions for *cancellations* and *broken appointments.*

Cancellations are defined as patients who inform you of a missed appointment prior to the scheduled visit.

Broken appointments are defined as patients who do not inform you that they will not keep their appointment prior to the scheduled time.

		W	S
1. Have the procedures for scheduling patients been explained to all responsible individual(s)?	2 Yes 0 No X	8	=
2. Are your scheduling policies and procedures in writing?	2 Yes 0 No X	4	=
3. Do you have a follow-up system for cancelled appointments?	2 Yes 0 No X	6	=
4. Do you have a follow-up system for broken appointments?	2 Yes 0 No X	5	=
5. Do you have a short notice call list of patients to fill in cancelled appointments?	2 Yes 0 No X	6	=
6. Do you plan procedures in advance for your patient's next visit?	2 Yes 0 No X	7	=

APPOINTMENT SCHEDULING WORKSHEET—cont'd

			W	S

7. Do you require that all appointments be confirmed?

   2 Yes
   0 No   X 3 =

8. Are you aware of all changes in
   the daily schedule?

   2 Yes
   0 No   X 4 =

9. Do you set aside buffer time for
   emergency patients?

   2 Yes
   0 No   X 6 =

10. Do you follow up on patients
    who cancel?

    2 Yes
    0 No   X 6 =

11. Do you keep a daily record of
    the number of patients who
    cancel appointments?

    2 Yes
    0 No   X 3 =

12. Do you record on the patient's
    chart each time an appointment
    is cancelled?

    2 Yes
    0 No   X 8 =

13. Do you keep a daily record of
    broken appointments?

    2 Yes
    0 No   X 3 =

14. Do you follow up broken ap-
    pointments?

    2 Yes
    0 No   X 5 =

15. Do you record on the patient's
    chart each time an appointment
    is broken?

    2 Yes
    0 No   X 9 =

Total _____

3 Recall program analysis

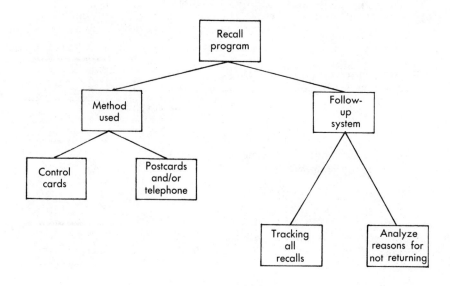

A key to continued success in your practice is a well-run recall program. The critical features of any effective recall program are that it be simple, require a minimum of administrative procedures, and provide maximum motivation for the patient. A well-run recall system can provide a practice with 20% to 30% of its annual gross production, provide a new source of patients, and provide a source of further treatment for existing patients. Because the competition for existing patients remains strong for most practices today, every effort must be made to retain those patients who have completed treatment and are to be seen for maintenance and/or have delayed a phase of their treatment plan for economic or other reasons. In addition, one of the best referral sources for new patients is your existing patient pool. If your recall program loses a percentage of patients yearly because of the lack of proper follow-up, you also have lost the opportunity for those patients to refer new patients to your practice. In almost all instances, poor patient follow-up can be avoided by the development of a recall program that can track each patient effectively and will not ''lose'' your patient unless you make an informed decision to delete him or her from your patient rolls.

The key factors of the recall program (shown in the diagram above) are the method used and the follow-up system. There are basically three types of recall methods: the advance appointment, the written reminder, and the telephone recall. Most practices do not use one method exclusively but rather use a combination of them. The primary problem with most recall programs is the follow-up system. This is usually attributed to the inadequate monitoring of patients to be scheduled for recalls and the careless follow-up of patients who were scheduled for recall but did not make or keep an appointment.

Your follow-up system should be able to determine the reasons why recall appointments are not being made or kept, locate and contact patients who have not responded to recall notices, and determine the reasons patients are not returning to your practice. Your recall program should therefore include a reporting format that allows you to determine very quickly the proportion of patients who respond to recall. Thus the impact of a new practice in your area may be readily examined with the use of recall information reports.

•   •   •

To assess the effectiveness of your recall program, please answer all questions on the recall program worksheets. If you cannot answer all the questions yourself, ask your receptionist and/or dental hygienist to assist you. If you score less that 104, refer to the recall program recommendations on p. 58.

RECALL PROGRAM ANALYSIS WORKSHEET

Directions: Answer each question by circling the appropriate response. Multiply the weight (W) for each question in the left column by the value of your response, Yes = 2, No = 0. Add the totals in the right-hand column to determine your score (S) for this section.

			W	S

1. Do you follow a written recall procedure? 　　2 Yes 　0 No 　X 　| 4 = |

2. Do you use a recall control card for each patient? 　　2 Yes 　0 No 　X 　| 8 = |

3. Do you use a log or recall control card to follow up on patients who have not scheduled an appointment or have missed their scheduled appointment? 　　2 Yes 　0 No 　X 　| 9 = |

4. If patients are supposed to contact the office to schedule a recall appointment and do not, do you contact them? 　　2 Yes 　0 No 　X 　| 9 = |

5. Do you contact patients at least two times if they do not respond to any recall messages? 　　2 Yes 　0 No 　X 　| 4 = |

6. Does each patient who comes in for a recall appointment receive a thorough dental examination by the doctor? 　　2 Yes 　0 No 　X 　| 6 = |

7. Are all patients who complete nonemergency treatment automatically placed in the recall system? 　　2 Yes 　0 No 　X 　| 7 = |

8. Do you know on a monthly basis the percentage of recalls that do not return to your practice? 　　2 Yes 　0 No 　X 　| 5 = |

RECALL PROGRAM ANALYSIS WORKSHEET—cont'd

W   S

9. Do you analyze reasons why patients on recall do not return to your practice?　2 Yes　0 No　**X**　| 4 = |

10. Is health education a planned component of your recall system?　2 Yes　0 No　**X**　| 5 = |

Total _____

4 Personnel management

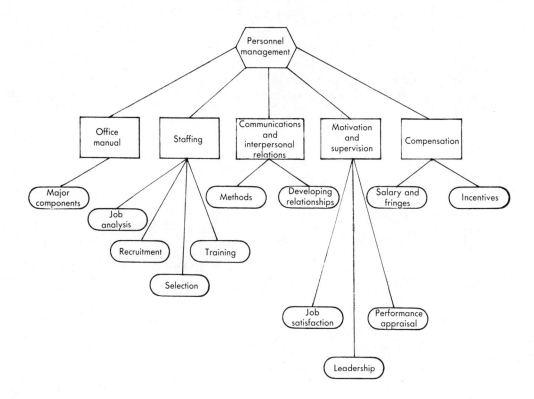

The most challenging and time-consuming aspect of managing a dental practice is managing people. Over the years a tremendous amount of research has been done in business and industry examining such areas as leadership styles, effective communications methods, the development of interpersonal relationships, the motivation of employees, the measurement of staff performance, and the supervision of personnel. All of these areas and more are applicable to your dental practice in varying degrees, depending on the size of your staff and your management style. The key factors involved in personnel management include developing and maintaining an office manual, staffing, establishing effective communications, and establishing sound policies of motivation and compensation (see diagram above).

The office manual is the source document for all policies and procedures that must be developed in every practice. All aspects of your practice operations, including every area related to managing personnel, should be described in writing and included in your office manual. Although it is admittedly a time-consuming project, the development of a comprehensive office manual will contribute to consistent job performance, increased staff productivity and reduced stress levels.

Staffing consists of numerous processes, each of which must be completed in a precise manner to ensure that you find the right person for the right job in your practice. Not only is it important in staffing to select the right person, but it is also important to bring that person into the practice in a way that will ensure an effective performance in the shortest possible time. An overview of staffing appears in Fig. 5.

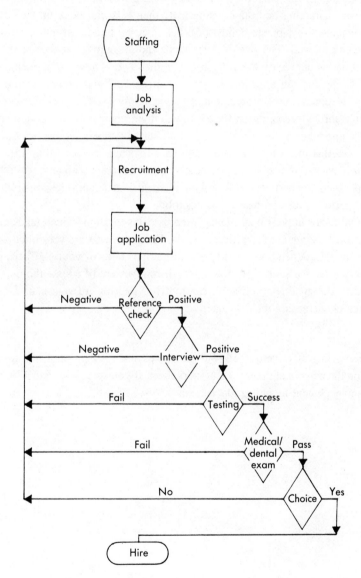

Fig. 5. Staffing overview.

The lack of effective communications between the doctor and the staff and among staff members is a major cause of problems in many practices. Communication is the primary method of developing and maintaining effective interpersonal relationships. Proper coordination of the staff cannot occur without the practice of appropriate communication skills. Communication also implies feedback and establishing a climate in which feedback can occur. Many times staff members in a busy practice never seem able to discuss problems, which can result in a crisis when tempers boil. Communication can be formalized in your practice by conducting regularly scheduled staff meetings. The manner in which meetings are conducted is equally important to ensure concrete actions. The staff's access to you is a key element for creating a climate in which problems can be discussed before they disrupt efficient practice operations.

Ensuring that people perform the job they were hired to do is a common problem for many dentists. Directing and supervising staff members can be a time-consuming yet necessary responsibility for the dentist or office manager and is essential if your practice goals are to be achieved. The size of the practice and the number of staff members have a direct effect on the degree of supervision required. As you know, some members of your staff seem to get the job done under any circumstances, and others require additional supervision, feedback, or reinforcement. Motivating your staff can be achieved in many ways, such as through recognition for a job well done, increased pay, or job enrichment. It is equally important to recognize that not all staff members require the same type of motivation and that motivational needs may vary for the same person at different times. *Supervision* is the act of overseeing, of watching and directing with authority, the work of others. Supervision consists of the following elements: leadership, responsibility and task delegation, performance appraisal, and discipline.

The final factor in personnel management is compensation, which takes many forms beyond the direct payment of salaries or wages. Fringe benefits are very important to most workers today and, depending on the age and marital status of your staff, fringe benefits can be a very effective source of motivation. Incentives are of course the purest form of reward and, if designed appropriately, can motivate and reward your staff for improving performance or increasing their productivity.

• • •

To assess the effectiveness of your personnel management policies, answer all the questions on the personnel management worksheet. If you score less than 188, refer to the personnel management recommendations on p. 59.

PERSONNEL MANAGEMENT WORKSHEET

Directions: Answer each question by circling the appropriate response. Multiply the weight (W) for each question in the left column by the value of your response, Yes = 2, No = 0. Add the totals in the right-hand column to determine your score (S) for this section.

W   S

1. Do you have written personnel policies? 2 Yes 0 No X 5 =

2. Do you review your office manual at least every 6 months? 2 Yes 0 No X 2 =

3. Do you have written job descriptions? 2 Yes 0 No X 5 =

4. Are your job descriptions reviewed at least annually? 2 Yes 0 No X 7 =

5. When hiring staff, do you check references? 2 Yes 0 No X 6 =

6. Are all candidates asked the same set of specific questions in the interview? 2 Yes 0 No X 5 =

7. Do you have a probationary period for new employees? 2 Yes 0 No X 7 =

8. Are new employees assigned to someone who will orient them to their job in the practice? 2 Yes 0 No X 7 =

PERSONNEL MANAGEMENT WORKSHEET—cont'd

			W	S

9. Do you have a formal training program for new staff members?

2 Yes
0 No

X 3 =

10. Do you conduct staff meetings at least once each month?

2 Yes
0 No

X 4 =

11. Do you conduct formal, written performance evaluations for your staff members at least annually?

2 Yes
0 No

X 8 =

12. On which of the following do you base raises for your staff?
   a. Performance evaluation

2 Yes
0 No

X 4 =

   b. Cost of living

2 Yes
0 No

X 2 =

   c. Staff expectations

2 Yes
0 No

X 1 =

   d. Whether you can afford it

2 Yes
0 No

X -1 =

   e. Length of service

2 Yes
0 No

X -1 =

   f. Outside salary competition

2 Yes
0 No

X 1 =

PERSONNEL MANAGEMENT WORKSHEET—cont'd

13. Which of the following incentives do you use to motivate your staff?

    a. Salary increases

        2 Yes
        0 No   X

        W   S
        2 =

    b. Recognition of achievement (e.g., regularly compliment performance)

        2 Yes
        0 No   X   8 =

    c. Increased responsibility and authority

        2 Yes
        0 No   X   4 =

    d. Monetary performance incentives (e.g., bonus for reaching specific goals)

        2 Yes
        0 No   X   3 =

    e. Increased fringe benefits (e.g., educational opportunities)

        2 Yes
        0 No   X   4 =

14. Do you invite your staff to participate in making decisions?

        2 Yes
        0 No   X   6 =

15. Do you know the limitations of your state's dental practice act regarding the delegation of duties to auxiliaries?

        2 Yes
        0 No   X   6 =

16. Do you delegate as much as possible within state dental practice act limitations?

        2 Yes
        0 No   X   4 =

PERSONNEL MANAGEMENT WORKSHEET—cont'd

17. Do you encourage and use staff
    suggestions?

    2 Yes
    0 No

    X

    W   S

    6 =

18. Do you encourage your staff to
    consult with you when they have
    have questions or problems con-
    cerning their job?

    2 Yes
    0 No

    X

    5 =

    Total _____

5 Inventory system analysis

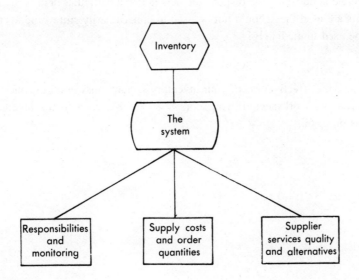

Many dentists do not develop a system for inventory control in their practice. Although inventory control is not the largest component of practice overhead, the development of an inventory control system can provide significant savings in cash as well as physical space. The goal of any inventory system is to provide an accurate report of available supplies and to indicate when supplies should be purchased. Nothing can be more frustrating than to realize a particular item is out of stock in the middle of a clinical procedure. Equally frustrating is to discover that a large supply of your materials are outdated and cannot be used. Both problems can definitely be avoided through the development of an inventory control system. The overview of an inventory system appears in the diagram above.

The first step in establishing your inventory system is to allocate to one individual the responsibility for developing and maintaining it. It is essential to know the reorder time for each supply and its respective source. This information is easily recorded on a master index file card. Of equal importance are determining the utilization rate of each item and calculating the reorder point for contacting the supplier. It is also advantageous to list a secondary supplier for emergency situations.

Physical space requirements in your practice may affect your ability to bulk-order certain supplies or to save cash by taking advantage of discounts. On the other hand, if any bulk-ordered items have a definite shelf life and their utilization rate is slower than the shelf life, dollars can be lost by discarding nonusable items. Every one in the practice must cooperate in notifying the responsible person that a particular item is running low. If mobile carts are used they should not be used to unnecessarily store supplies that are not going to be used immediately.

•   •   •

To assess the effectiveness of your inventory system, answer all the questions on the inventory analysis worksheet. If you score less than 83, refer to the inventory recommendations on p. 60.

INVENTORY WORKSHEET

Directions: Answer each question by circling the appropriate response. Multiply the weight (W) for each question in the left column by the value of your response, Yes = 2, No = 0. Add the totals in the right-hand column to determine your score (S) for this section.

				W	S
1.	Have the procedures for monitoring and ordering inventory been explained to all responsible individuals?	2 Yes 0 No	X	8	=
2.	Is only one individual responsible for ordering the majority of your supplies?	2 Yes 0 No	X	5	=
3.	Which of the following steps do you use to monitor inventory flow? a. Keep a master list posted in the storage area indicating the reorder point for each item.	2 Yes 0 No	X	1	=
	b. Label the shelves in the supply closet with the product name and reorder time.	2 Yes 0 No	X	1	=
	c. Attach a tag to supplies at the reorder point.	2 Yes 0 No	X	3	=
	d. Attach a special indicator to items that have a shelf life.	2 Yes 0 No	X	2	=
	e. Check off items on a master list when the reorder point is reached.	2 Yes 0 No	X	1	=
	f. Check the master list on a scheduled basis.	2 Yes 0 No	X	1	=

INVENTORY WORKSHEET—cont'd

W   **S**

4. Do you know how far in advance   2 Yes
   to order from each supplier?   0 No   X $\boxed{9 =}$

5. Do you have a supplier who can   2 Yes
   be called for emergency situa-   0 No   X $\boxed{4 =}$
   tions?

6. Do you use a follow-up log or con- 2 Yes
   trol card to monitor supplies on   0 No   X $\boxed{6 =}$
   order?

7. Do you follow up on orders that   2 Yes
   have not been received on their   0 No   X $\boxed{8 =}$
   scheduled arrival date?

8. Did supplies with a limited shelf 2 Yes
   life need to be discarded more   0 No   X $\boxed{-2 =}$
   than two times during the past
   year?

9. Did you run out of supplies more 2 Yes
   than three times during the past 0 No   X $\boxed{-2 =}$
   year?

Total _____

6 Laboratory flow analysis

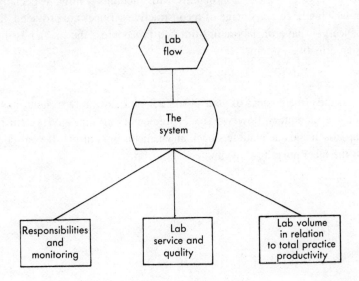

How many times during the past year have you been embarrassed because a laboratory case did not arrive on time for your patient's appointment? Ask yourself how many times the laboratory did not trim your dies properly; set your denture correctly; return the castings you requested, but rather sent a finished crown; or did not have a case ready when promised. These pitfalls and stress producers in your practice can be reduced through the development of a laboratory flow system. The relationship between you and your laboratory(ies) is of utmost importance, especially from the perspectives of quality and timeliness. The laboratory flow system is depicted in the diagram above.

The first major factor for your laboratory flow system is to develop a laboratory case monitoring system that must contain the following: a master log (containing the date a case is sent, the date a case is promised, and the date a case is received) and a tickler system (showing the date cases are expected). Assigning this responsibility to one individual is necessary to avoid any breakdown in follow-up between your practice and the laboratory.

The next factor involves the quality of workmanship. If you are constantly arguing with your laboratory over their product or the processes they use to give you that final product, perhaps you are (1) not communicating your requests and demands clearly or (2) using a laboratory that is inferior to the standards of acceptability that you have set. Each practice has a varying degree of problems with laboratory flow, especially in those instances in which a large percentage of reconstructive services are provided. The greater the dependence you have on laboratory-finished procedures, the greater is the need for developing an effective system.

• • •

To assess the effectiveness of your practice's laboratory flow system, answer all the questions on the laboratory flow worksheet, remembering that any system requires an organized approach and adequate feedback mechanisms or controls. If you score less than 75, refer to the laboratory flow recommendations on p. 60.

LABORATORY FLOW WORKSHEET

Directions: Answer each question by circling the appropriate response. Multiply the weight (W) for each question in the left column by the value of your response, Yes = 2, No = 0. Add the totals in the right-hand column to determine your score (S) for this section.

W   S

1. Have the procedures for monitoring laboratory flow been explained to all responsible individuals?   2 Yes   0 No   X $8 =$

2. Are all laboratory procedures in writing?   2 Yes   0 No   X $2 =$

3. Do you require that all laboratory case arrivals be confirmed?   2 Yes   0 No   X $5 =$

4. Do you require confirmation from the laboratory for the completion date of each case?   2 Yes   0 No   X $2 =$

5. Do you keep a master log on the due dates for cases?   2 Yes   0 No   X $7 =$

6. Do you review the master log daily?   2 Yes   0 No   X $6 =$

7. Do you use a file for duplicate laboratory authorizations filed under the date that the case is expected from the lab?   2 Yes   0 No   X $7 =$

8. Do you review daily the file of duplicate laboratory authorizations?   2 Yes   0 No   X $6 =$

LABORATORY FLOW WORKSHEET—cont'd

		W	**S**

9. Do you indicate by the patient's name in the appointment book the date the laboratory case is needed?   2 Yes
0 No   **X** | 2 = |

10. Do you know how many days the laboratory requires for each procedure?   2 Yes
0 No   **X** | 8 = |

Total _____

7 Bookkeeping/accounting system analysis

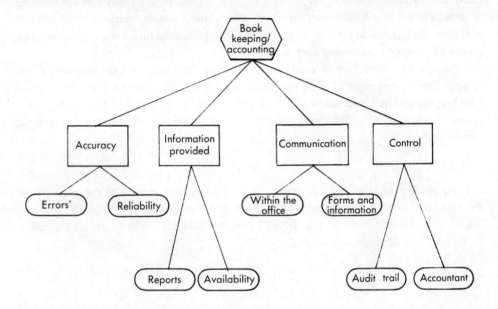

The proper recording of patients' fees and their timely collection are the major objectives of your bookkeeping system. Whether you use a manual system, a service bureau, or an in-house computer, your bookkeeping/accounting system must provide you with accurate and easily retrievable information. The major factors of an effective bookkeeping system are depicted in the diagram above.

Any system you use must be accurate and reliable. In the manual pegboard system, errors are minimized because entries are only made one time. The ability to write account information on patient's ledger cards, statements, and transaction slip are the major advantages of the one-write systems. Any effective bookkeeping system must also provide summary reports that allow the dentist to monitor the financial transactions of the practice. For example, reports of dentist/hygienist revenue and productivity should be available. This allows you to monitor your production on a daily and weekly basis. The information from most bookkeeping/accounting systems will also monitor expenses. A pegboard system, for example, can be converted into your practice's "checkbook." Your check amounts are then placed in predetermined expense categories that, when combined with your revenue information, provide you with an income and expense report. Service bureaus and in-house computer systems can perform essentially the same functions as manual systems.

In any bookkeeping system, proper communication between the system, the patient, the doctor, and the staff member working with that system must be maintained. Thus a transmittal form is required that will list charges, communicate outstanding balances, and show payment for the procedure. With a pegboard system, a buck slip is a working part of the system. Service bureaus differ as to the method of data entry, namely batch processing or direct entry into a remote terminal. With an in-house system, entries can be directly made into the terminal at the time of the actual visit or recorded on a buck slip that is batch processed at some time during each workday.

Adequate controls must be established and maintained to protect the integrity of any system. The development of audit trails and checkpoints must be incorporated into any bookkeeping system. Your accountant's responsibility in this area will help to develop a system that will prevent dishonesty and alleviate the possibility of temptation to beat the system.

•   •   •

To assess your existing bookkeeping/accounting system, answer all the questions on the bookkeeping/accounting worksheet. If you cannot answer all the questions yourself, ask your receptionist to assist you. If you score less than 112, refer to the bookkeeping/accounting recommendations on p. 61.

BOOKKEEPING/ACCOUNTING WORKSHEET

Directions: Answer each question by circling the appropriate response. Multiply the weight (W) for each question in the left column by the value of your response, Yes = 2, No = 0. Add the totals in the right-hand column to determine your score (S) for this section.

	W	S

1. Have the responsible individuals been formally trained in the use of your bookkeeping system?   2 Yes / 0 No   **X** | 6 = |

2. Does your system provide a mechanism to check for errors?   2 Yes / 0 No   **X** | 9 = |

3. Do you use a written communication (e.g., a buck slip) between the operatory and the person responsible for making the entry into the bookkeeping system?   2 Yes / 0 No   **X** | 6 = |

4. Does your system include the following?
   a. Numbered transaction slips   2 Yes / 0 No   **X** | 1 = |

   b. A recording of all treatment transactions   2 Yes / 0 No   **X** | 1 = |

   c. A recording of all charges   2 Yes / 0 No   **X** | 2 = |

   d. A recording of all payments   2 Yes / 0 No   **X** | 2 = |

   e. Proof or a check of each day's transaction   2 Yes / 0 No   **X** | 3 = |

BOOKKEEPING/ACCOUNTING WORKSHEET—cont'd

W   S

f. An account ledger card   2 Yes
                                 0 No   **X** | 1 = |

5. Which of the following features does your manual or automated bookkeeping system provide?
   a. Account by individual or family   2 Yes / 0 No **X** | 1 = |

   b. Charge for treatment   2 Yes / 0 No **X** | 2 = |

   c. Total balance   2 Yes / 0 No **X** | 2 = |

   d. Balance owed by the patient   2 Yes / 0 No **X** | 1 = |

   e. Balance owed by a third party   2 Yes / 0 No **X** | 1 = |

6. What information is provided by your bookkeeping/accounting system?
   a. Total accounts receivable balance for practice   2 Yes / 0 No **X** | 3 = |

   b. Aging of total accounts receivable   2 Yes / 0 No **X** | 1 = |

BOOKKEEPING/ACCOUNTING WORKSHEET—cont'd

c. Production of insurance forms   2 Yes   0 No   **X**   **W** **S** | 1 = |

d. Billing   2 Yes   0 No   **X** | 2 = |

e. Income/production reports   2 Yes   0 No   **X** | 1 = |

f. Expense reports   2 Yes   0 No   **X** | 1 = |

g. Financial statements   2 Yes   0 No   **X** | 1 = |

7. Does your accountant or system provide you with at least quarterly income statements?   2 Yes   0 No   **X** | 7 = |

8. Do you periodically check for the accuracy of entries into the system?   2 Yes   0 No   **X** | 7 = |

9. Does your accountant periodically review the accuracy of entries   2 Yes   0 No   **X** | 4 = |

Total _____

8 Practice building

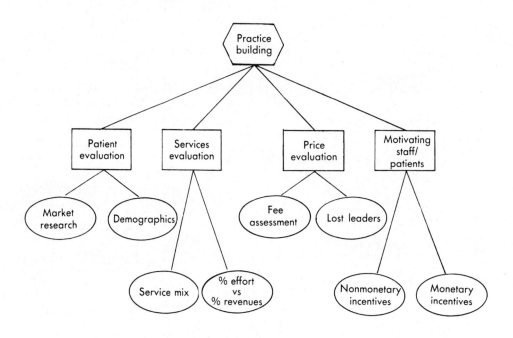

It is not uncommon for general practitioners and specialists to lament that their productivity is decreasing or leveling off. The dental literature in the past few years has contained many articles on ways to help you increase your patient load or prevent your regular patients from leaving your practice. Commonly referred to as practice building, this area of dental practice management is more accurately termed marketing and communication concepts. The true emphasis on marketing should not merely be the gimmicks you can use to attract new or retain existing patients. Rather it should consist of an organized and systematic approach that describes your patients and analyzes why they continue to return to your practice.

Practice building or marketing consists of several key factors as depicted in the diagram above. Knowing your patients is a critical factor. Through simple marketing research techniques, your practice can be segmented into major patient groupings by socioeconomic status, age, and geographic location. Your goals are to understand the market from which the majority of your patients come and the reasons they return to you after the completion of regular treatment. That is why an effective recall system is so essential. Knowing the reasons those patients return on a regular basis can give you the data necessary to attract those types of patients as new patients for your practice. It is also important to know your strengths and to identify your particular competitive advantage. Such factors as your personality, your competent and friendly staff, a comfortable office, and convenient operating hours can help to give you that competitive edge. It is your responsibility to discover from your patients, especially those on recall, which factors apply.

The next factor is product evaluation. Throughout this workbook, productivity analysis and management have been emphasized, and practice building is no exception. Analyzing these services in which you spend the most time and correlating them to those services that generate the greatest proportion of revenue are the two major components of evaluating your ''product.'' For example, if you are spending 30% of your time on a service that only generates 8% of your total revenue, it is obvious that a change must be made. You must either reduce the time spent on that service or increase your fees. Analyzing services that are more profitable and searching for strategies that will increase the number of these services is another component of this process.

The third factor is the review of all fees on a regular basis. Perhaps your fees are too high in comparison with similar dental practices in your area. Some downward readjustment may be necessary if you can determine from those patients who are not returning to your practice that their primary reason was high fees. Obviously your professional time and services are worth a fair fee, but unnecessarily high fees may deter new patients from entering your practice. The use of a ''loss leader'' is still an excellent idea, provided that you can demonstrate that a service or group of services that are not truly profitable will generate additional services for you and bring patients to the practice. Good examples of loss leaders are examination fees and prophylaxis.

Finally, motivating your staff and present patients to bring new patients to your practice is a key factor that is often overlooked. Both groups know you well and can very easily serve as public relations representatives for your practice. Merely thanking them for bringing in new patients may not be sufficient. Instead, providing them with incentives may be the answer.

• • •

To assess the effectiveness of your practice building approach, please answer all questions on the practice building worksheet. If you score less than 194, refer to the practice building recommendations on p. 61.

PRACTICE BUILDING WORKSHEET

Directions: Answer each question by circling the appropriate response. Multiply the weight (W) for each question in the left column by the value of your response, Yes = 2, No = 0. Add the totals in the right-hand column to determine your score (S) for this section. In addition, please write answers to those questions that require written responses.

1. Can you list the five procedures that contribute to most of your practice production? Please list them, showing their appropriate percentage of total production.

W	S
2 Yes	
0 No **X**	**4** =

Service	% of total practice production
_____	_____ %
_____	_____ %
_____	_____ %
_____	_____ %
_____	_____ %

2. Were the procedures on which you spent the most time the top five revenue producers?

   2 Yes
   0 No   **X**   **7** =

3. Do you have a system that identifies your sources of new patients?

   2 Yes
   0 No   **X**   **8** =

4. Do you have a zipcode breakdown for all of your active patients?

   2 Yes
   0 No   **X**   **4** =

5. Have you asked patients to refer new patients to you during the last year?

   2 Yes
   0 No   **X**   **3** =

PRACTICE BUILDING WORKSHEET—cont'd

| | | | | W | S |

6. Have you contacted medical professionals in your community regarding the services that your practice provides within the past year?
2 Yes
0 No
X [2] =

7. Do you participate in study clubs on a regular basis?
2 Yes
0 No
X [2] =

8. Do you prepare comprehensive treatment plans?
2 Yes
0 No
X [5] =

9. Do you schedule formal case presentation sessions?
2 Yes
0 No
X [4] =

10. Do you know the reasons why your patients do not accept your treatment plans?
2 Yes
0 No
X [5] =

11. Are fees discussed before starting treatment?
2 Yes
0 No
X [7] =

12. Are you doing the following in your practice?
a. Sending welcome letters to new patients
2 Yes
0 No
X [2] =

b. Sending thank you letters for referrals
2 Yes
0 No
X [3] =

c. Calling patients who may have some discomfort from treatment
2 Yes
0 No
X [4] =

PRACTICE BUILDING WORKSHEET—cont'd

			W	S

d. Using patient surveys   2 Yes
                                 0 No   **X** | 1 = |

e. Sending cards for special   2 Yes
    events   0 No   **X** | 1 = |

f. Sending patient newsletters 2 Yes
                                 0 No   **X** | 1 = |

13. Do you have a patient brochure?   2 Yes
                                      0 No   **X** | 4 = |

14. Do you have a formal patient   2 Yes
    education program?   0 No   **X** | 4 = |

15. Do you follow up on your recalls?   2 Yes
                                        0 No   **X** | 8 = |

16. Do you know the demographic   2 Yes
    characteristics of your patient   0 No   **X** | 3 = |
    population (e.g., age, sex, socio-
    economic status)?

17. Do you know the demographic   2 Yes
    characteristics of the area you   0 No   **X** | 3 = |
    serve?

18. Do you know the direct costs for   2 Yes
    each of the services that you pro-   0 No   **X** | 5 = |
    vide?

PRACTICE BUILDING WORKSHEET—cont'd

			W	S

19. Are your fees based on costs?   2 Yes
                                      0 No   X | 5 = |

20. Are your fees based on a per-
    ceived patient demand basis?   2 Yes
                                      0 No   X | 3 = |

21. Do you provide incentives for
    patients who refer new patients   2 Yes
    to your practice?   0 No   X | 3 = |

22. Are your operating hours based   2 Yes
    on patient demand?   0 No   X | 6 = |

23. Do you compensate your staff
    for generating new patients for   2 Yes
    the practice?   0 No   X | 4 = |

24. Do you know why patients do   2 Yes
    not return to your practice?   0 No   X | 4 = |

25. Do you know how many dentists   2 Yes
    serve the people living within   0 No   X | 3 = |
    3 miles of your office?

Total _____

9 Financial management

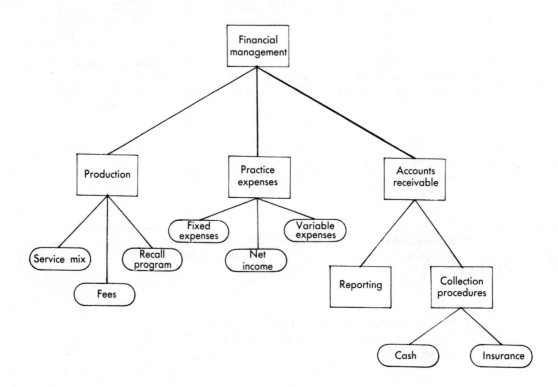

Are you satisfied with the direction of your practice's financial status? Do you know the relationship of your production to your overhead? More specifically, what can you do to control expenses and increase production? A necessary first step in answering these questions is to develop a financial management system that can provide you with easily accessible information concerning your production, expenses, and accounts receivable. The relationships of these factors is diagrammed above.

Adequate production depends primarily on three factors: available patients, practice efficiency, and available dentist/hygienist hours. Patient availability is the most difficult factor to control. This, of course, depends on such variables as the way in which you market your practice, your competition with similar practices, and your current practice location. The available number of dentist hours is directly controllable and is based on your personal work habits and preferences for leisure time and life-style. Practice efficiency can be directly controlled by efficient office design, the use of assistants, effective appointment/scheduling policies, your personal work habits, the standardization of all procedures, and a well-trained staff. It is important in production management to analyze your past performance, to set new goals, and to achieve them. The emphasis on increased productivity must also be shared by all staff members, both care providers and auxiliaries.

Another aspect of office production is your service mix. You probably have a preference for performing certain clinical procedures. Also, not all services you provide are truly profitable. Therefore being able to analyze your production by segmenting it into service areas (such as operative or crown and bridge) provides you with an analysis of the time you are spending with your patients. It also will aid you in determining if those services that you are primarily providing your patients are truly your most profitable. If not, you may have to seriously review a portion of your fee schedule.

A review of fees must be undertaken on a routine basis because often your desired productivity goal may not be achieved without raising fees, if all other actions to increase patient flow, cut expenses, and increase efficiency have been taken. Fees are similar to any other prices for goods and services in the economy in that they reflect the cost of providing services to your patients. A review and appropriate revision of fees should be done often so that the absolute changes in fees will be smaller, and therefore more acceptable to patients, than the larger fee changes made necessary by infrequent reviews.

The analysis of expenses and how they may directly or indirectly influence production is another major factor. Staff salaries and fringe benefits usually comprise the largest portion of practice overhead, but your staff members are the most important resource for achieving your desired goals of increased productivity. Some fine tuning of other practice expenses, such as laboratory expenses and supplies, can also be achieved. Instituting an effective inventory control system, some careful bulk ordering, and increasing your staff's awareness of waste can help to reduce your dental supplies overhead. Shopping around for a lower cost per unit between laboratories, without sacrificing quality, may aid in trimming your laboratory expenses.

Another major impact on office productivity is the effectiveness of your recall system. Since an efficient recall system can contribute 20% to 30% of your total practice revenues, and since it serves as a constant source of new patient referrals, much attention should be given to this area. As you recall, this was discussed thoroughly in Chapter 3.

The third major factor in financial management is accounts receivable. The timely collection of fees and the processing of insurance claims are critical to the cash flow management of most practices today. The important aspects of effective collection procedures were presented in Chapter 1.

• • •

To assess the effectiveness of your financial management, complete the financial management worksheet. If you score less than the score indicated for each section, refer to the financial management recommendations on p. 63.

FINANCIAL MANAGEMENT WORKSHEET

Directions: Complete this worksheet by checking the appropriate response or computing the required calculations.

1. Did you establish goals for increased production from last year to this year?

   Yes _____

   No _____

   a. Were your goals met?

   Yes _____

   No _____

2. Can you calculate the percent of change in your total practice production (including the hygienist's production) from last year until this year?

   Yes _____

   No _____

   a. Calculation of changes in production:

   List the total production for this year (a) = $ _____
   List the total production for last year (b) = $ _____

   STEP I: Calculation of change in production (C)

   $C = a - b$
   $C = $ _____

   STEP II: Calculation of percent of change in production (P)

   $P = \dfrac{C}{b}$

   $P = $ _____

   STEP III: If your percent of change (P) is less than your established goal, refer to the financial management recommendations on p. 63.

3. Can you calculate the percent of change in your personal net income (before taxes) from last year to this year?

   Yes _____

   No _____

   a. Calculation of changes in your net income

   List your net income for this year   (d) = $ _____
   List your net income for last year   (e) = $ _____

   STEP I: Calculation of change in net income (I)

   $I = d - e$
   $I = $ _____

   STEP II: Calculation of percent of change in net income (N)

   $N = \dfrac{I}{e}$

   $N = $ _____

   STEP III: If your percent of change (N) is less than your established goal, refer to the financial management recommendations on p. 63.

FINANCIAL MANAGEMENT WORKSHEET—cont'd

4. Can you calculate the percent of change in your hourly production from last year to this year?

Yes _____

No _____

   a. Calculation of change in hourly production

      List the number of hours you had available to see patients this year
         (f) = _____ hours

      List the number of hours you had available to see patients last year
         (g) = _____ hours

       STEP I: Determine the hourly production for this year (R) (refer to No. 2a)

$$R = \frac{a}{f}$$

       STEP II: Determine the hourly production from last year (S) (refer to No. 2a)

$$S = \frac{b}{g}$$

       STEP III: Calculation of change in production per hour (T) from year to year

$$T = R - S$$
$$T = \text{_____}$$

       STEP IV: Calculation of percent of change in production per hour from last year to this year (V)

$$V = \frac{T}{S}$$
$$V = \text{_____}$$

       STEP V: If your percent of change in production per hour (V) is negative or less than your established goal, refer to the financial management recommendations on p. 63.

FINANCIAL MANAGEMENT WORKSHEET—cont'd

5. Can you calculate the percent of changes in your major expense categories from this year to last year?   Yes _____   No _____

   a. List by percent of expenses your overhead from last year and this year.

Percent of production

Description	(X) Last year	(Y) This year	(W) Acceptable ranges (%)
Salary/wages (not including yourself or associates)	____%	____%	12-19
Employee benefits	____%	____%	1-3
Occupancy (include rent, lease/mortgage, utilities, and janitorial service)	____%	____%	4-10
Laboratory charges	____%	____%	9-17
Dental supplies (include drugs and office)	____%	____%	4-9
Practice-related insurance (include malpractice insurance)	____%	____%	1-2
Professional expenses (dues/ subscriptions, continuing education costs, travel to meetings, etc.)	____%	____%	1-2
Legal and professional fees	____%	____%	1-3
Taxes on business property	____%	____%	1-3
Interest on business indebtedness	____%	____%	1-3
Repairs	____%	____%	0-2
Depreciation	____%	____%	2-4
Marketing	____%	____%	0-10
Total expenses	____%	____%	45-70

STEP I: Calculate the change in practice expenses from year to year (Q)

$$Q = Y - X$$
$$Q = \text{_____}$$

STEP II: Calculate the percent of change in practice expenses from year to year (U)

$$U = \frac{Q}{X} \times 100\%$$

STEP III: If your percent of change is greater than 8%, refer to the financial management recommendations on p. 63.

STEP IV: If any of the individual expense percentages entered in column Y (this year's expenses) are outside the range shown, refer to the financial management recommendations on p. 63.

FINANCIAL MANAGEMENT WORKSHEET—cont'd

6. Do you know the percentage of recalls that do not return to your practice on a monthly basis?

Yes _____

No _____

STEP I: List the number of monthly recall notices (appointments that should be made) sent for the past 6 months and compare to the number of actual recall appointments seen during that same period.

Number of recalls that should be seen per month	Number of appointments seen	(Z) Percent seen
*1st month	*XXX	_____ %
2nd month	_____	_____ %
3rd month	_____	_____ %
4th month	_____	_____ %
5th month	_____	_____ %
6th month	_____	_____ %
7th month	_____	_____ %

•You cannot calculate the first month since you determine the number of appointments seen based on the number of recalls to be appointed in the prior month.

STEP II: Calculation of percent seen (Z)

$$Z = \frac{\text{Number of appointments seen}}{\text{Number of recalls that should be seen per month}}$$

a. Can you determine the reasons patients are not returning to your practice for their recall visits?

Yes _____

No _____

b. Does your staff try to determine the reasons patients do not return for their recall visit?

Yes _____

No _____

STEP I: If you answer no to questions 6a and 6b, refer to the recall recommendations on p. 58.

FINANCIAL MANAGEMENT WORKSHEET—cont'd

7. Can you determine the accounts receivable/collection ratio for the past 12 months?

Yes _____
No _____

   a. Can you determine the accounts receivable ratio for the past 6 months?

Yes _____
No _____

   STEP I: If you answer no to questions 7 and 7a, refer to the collections procedures recommendations on p. 55.

   b. Calculate the accounts receivable/collection ratios (account receivable turnover).

List	Past 12 months		Six months ago
Total collections	(i) _____	(k)	_____
Total accounts receivable	(j) _____	(l)	_____
Total production	(b) _____	(m)	_____

   STEP I: Calculate the accounts receivable turnover for last year (F)

$$F = \frac{j}{b}$$

   F = _____

   STEP II: If F is greater than 1.5, refer to the financial management recommendations on p. 63.

   STEP III: Calculate the accounts receivable turnover (O) for the prior 6 months.

$$O = \frac{l}{m}$$

   O = _____

   STEP IV: If O is greater than 1.5, refer to the financial management recommendations on p. 63.

   c. Calculate the collection/production ratio

   STEP I: Calculate the collection/production ratio for last year (L)

$$L = \frac{i}{a} \times 100\%$$

   L = _____

   STEP II: If L is less than 95%, refer to the financial management recommendations on p. 63.

10 Practice management recommendations

Now that you have completed your practice analysis worksheets, you may have discovered areas in which you scored below the established average. This chapter provides you with some recommendations that may improve your practice's performance in each practice management area. Remember, these recommendations are not the final answer. Rather they are suggestions that should start you in the right direction. Some of you may be able to follow these recommendations without additional help, but if your problem is a major one, you may require professional assistance in changing or improving that practice management area. Also keep in mind that any change, no matter how small, takes time and requires commitment from you and your staff to alter your habits. Proper follow-up is also needed to ensure that any changes become a permanent routine in your practice rather than a brief rallying point. Old habits have a way of returning in a few weeks or months without the proper reenforcement of those recommendations that you plan to implement.

COLLECTION PROCEDURES RECOMMENDATIONS

If you scored below 199 on the collection procedure worksheet, it would be helpful to review these recommendations. Some are very easy to implement; others will require considerable staff training and assistance from your accountant or management consultant. Some of these recommendations may be mutually exclusive because of the type of system you now use or the policies that you currently follow.

- Develop written collection policies to cover *at least*
    Initial office visit fee
    Payment of fee at time of treatment
    Use of finance charges
    Acceptance of assignment
    Copayment billing procedures
    Account billing cycle
    Follow-up procedure for past due accounts
    Use of collection agency and/or attorney
    Telephone guidelines for new patients as well as past due accounts
    Collection of emergency office visit fee
    Use of professional courtesy
    Use of bank cards (Visa and Mastercard)
    Use of payment/installment plans for expensive cases

- Train your staff in proper telephone procedures for collecting fees.
- Train your staff in techniques for collecting fees at the time of treatment
- Use a Truth in Lending form when appropriate.
- Inform all patients in writing of your practice's collection policies.
- Demand that all staff members and doctors adhere to office policies regarding collections.
- Provide a written receipt to any patient who pays cash.
- Send patient statements at a predetermined time(s) each month.
- Use a statement that has a professional appearance.
- Age all outstanding accounts according to the following categories
    - 0 to 30 days
    - 31 to 60 days
    - 61 to 90 days
    - 91 to 120 days
    - Over 120 days
- Use an accounts receivable aging report as a cash collection follow-up log. This should include the patient's business and residence telephone numbers.
- Record all conversations regarding delinquent accounts on the patient's record.
- Use an insurance follow-up log that includes the following information
    - Date of service
    - Date the claim is filed
    - Follow-up date
    - Patient's (insured's) name
    - Name of carrier and place to which claim is sent
    - Assignment (yes/no)
    - Amount of claim
    - Amount paid (date) and balance owed
- Make specific copayment arrangements prior to initiating treatment.
- Collect the copayment balance from the patient during the course of the treatment rather than after the claim has been paid.
- Consider a policy of not accepting assignment for cases less than a certain amount.
- Develop criteria for starting treatment without receiving preauthorization from the carrier.
- Develop a catalogue containing all current benefit plans for your patients.
- Establish a cycle for the completion and submission of claim forms. This should be completed at least weekly.
- Emphasize the use of credit cards when cash payment by a patient seems remote.
- Set deadlines for the receipt of a claim check in cases in which assignment has been accepted.
- Compute an accounts receivable total by insurance carrier on a monthly basis.
- Review the insurance log periodically to determine if your policies are being followed.
- Review the accounts receivable aging report at least monthly to monitor the progress of your collection procedures.

- Set goals by the percentage of aged accounts. For example
    0 to 30 days 50%
    30 to 60 days 40%
    60 to 90 days 10%
    Over 90 days 0%

APPOINTMENT SCHEDULING RECOMMENDATIONS

If you scored below 141, on the appointment scheduling worksheet, these recommendations on appointment scheduling and follow-up may prove to be helpful.

- Develop written policies that should at least include
    Handling of emergencies
    Protocol for scheduling routine patients
    Broken appointment and cancellation policies
    Time of day preference for performing certain procedures
    New patient information
    Handling concurrent care patients (specialists)
    Time length of appointments
    Recall policies
    Interfacing with the laboratory
- Calculate the average time required for most commonly performed services.
- Develop time units for most commonly performed services, such as one unit is equal to
    5 minutes
    10 minutes
    15 minutes
    20 minutes
- Enter a telephone number in the appointment book for all new patients.
- Enter a procedure code or an abbreviated name of the procedure beside each scheduled patient in the appointment book.
- Develop a definition of a true emergency and apply it to all patients who request an emergency appointment. Attempt to screen as many unnecessary emergencies as possible over the telephone.
- Try not to completely fill the appointment book for more than 3 to 4 weeks in advance to allow time for new patients.
- Schedule patients by operatory when using multiple operatories.
- Use color codes for more than one doctor.
- Develop a short-notice call list of patients for last minute broken appointments.
- Develop a master schedule for the appointment book at the beginning of each year with a monthly advance review of:
    Holidays when the practice will be closed
    Vacation days when the practice will be closed (for solos only)
    Continuing education course schedules
- Conduct periodic analyses of the times of day that patients demand first to get feedback regarding a possible change and/or expansion of office hours.

- Design an appointment sheet that allows you to extract at least the following information:

    New patients scheduled

    Recall patients scheduled

    Cancellations

    Broken appointments by type

    Emergencies

    Routine care patients

- Summarize on a weekly basis information regarding the type of patients scheduled (see the previous list).

- Use a transmittal slip that indicates the patient's balance, the charge, the next appointment date, and the length of the procedure(s) to be performed.

- Design a work schedule for each day and post it at various locations in the practice.

- Use buffer time (nonregularly scheduled time) to handle emergency situations, lateness, and delays in schedule.

RECALL PROGRAM RECOMMENDATIONS

If you scored below 104 on the recall program worksheet, it would be worthwhile to review these recommendations. An effective recall system is the major element for keeping your practice vital and in a growth mode. If you are a specialist, some of these recommendations may vary as to the frequency and type of recall appointment you will need in your practice.

- Develop a written recall policy to include

    System description

    Frequency of visits

    Follow-up procedures

    Analysis of monthly activity

- Schedule a recall appointment at the final hygiene visit.

- Use a recall control card for each patient.

- Provide patients with a confirmation postcard 2 weeks before their previously scheduled recall appointment, requesting that they schedule a recall appointment.

- Contact all patients who have not called to schedule a recall appointment by the first of the month. This is best done by telephone.

- Record notes of conversations when following up with recall patients.

- Place all recall control cards in an alphabetically ordered file by the month *before* their next recall appointment.

- Assess the reasons your patients are not returning for their recall visit. Telephone surveying is the most effective method of assessment.

- Develop monthly reports that include

    Number of patients to be scheduled for a recall appointment

    Number of recall visits actually scheduled

    Number of broken or cancelled recall appointments

    Number of patients who have delayed their recall appointment

    Number of recall patients who have left your practice. (Try to summarize major reasons, such as relocation.)

    Number of new patients referred by a patient on recall

PERSONNEL MANAGEMENT RECOMMENDATIONS

If you scored below 188 on the personnel management worksheet, it will be worth your time to review these recommendations. There may be some ideas included here that you never considered before. One fact is certain; any changes that you make regarding the managing of your personnel require time and effort. There are no quick fixes in personnel matters.

- Develop a policy and procedures manual that should include at least the following topics

  Introduction

      Philosophy of your practice

      Table of contents

      Purpose of the manual

      Goals and objectives of the practice

  Office policies

      Employment policies

      Policies governing employee conduct

      Duties of all employees

  Office procedures

      Business office procedures

      Patient treatment procedures

      Materials used in the office

      Equipment care and operation

  Inventory control
- Review job descriptions with all staff members at least annually.
- Develop written goals for each staff member.
- Schedule a performance review session for each staff member using a goal-oriented rating form.
- Review staff performance at least annually, but try to do so every 6 months.
- Establish a system for recruiting staff members to include:

  Advertising format and sources

  Screening by phone and/or resume

  Use of an employment application

  Standardized interview

  System for conducting reference checks

  Use of a rating sheet during interviews

  Involvement of key staff members in the interview process

  An induction program

  Placing a staff member in charge of training new staff
- Conduct frequent staff meetings using a prepared agenda often appointing a staff member as group leader
- Review salaries annually and try to provide raises at the same time each year.
- Develop performance-related criteria to increase salaries.
- Consider the use of monetary and nonmonetary incentives to reward staff members for exceptional performance.
- Make a conscious effort to be available to staff members for the discussion of office matters.

- Take corrective action immediately if someone is not doing his or her work.
- Try to thank your staff routinely and show appreciation for their doing a good job.
- Maintain an open line of communications with all staff members and encourage their feedback when appropriate.
- Analyze your work habits to see if some of your routine tasks can be delegated to someone else in the practice.
- Delegate tasks frequently and give the staff member adequate time and authority to complete the task.
- Avoid correcting a staff member in front of others, especially your patients.
- Develop a fringe benefit package that is competitive and addresses the majority of needs of your staff members.
- Remind your staff annually of their total compensation by calculating the amount of fringe benefits that you offer your staff and attach a summary to their W-2 forms in January of each year.

INVENTORY RECOMMENDATIONS

If you scored less than 83 on the inventory worksheet, please review the recommendations in this section. An inventory system is relatively inexpensive to install, and an effective system will save you money and reduce potential embarrassment if an item is unavailable when you need it.

- Assign the responsibility of controlling inventory as well as communicating with vendors to one person.
- Calculate your utilization of supplies and from that determine your reorder time.
- Determine the economic order quantity (EOQ) for each major supply item.
- List all supply items by reorder time or economic order quantity, vendor source(s), turnaround time, and the date the item was last ordered.
- Maintain a master list posted in the storage area indicating the reorder time or economic order quantity for each item.
- Use tags to indicate the reorder time or economic order quantity and their emergency order time.
- Review the master list on a regularly scheduled basis.
- Maintain a follow-up log or central card to monitor supplies on order.
- Analyze the discarding of supplies during the previous year because of limited shelf life.
- Develop a back-up list of vendors.

LABORATORY FLOW RECOMMENDATIONS

If you scored less than 75 on the laboratory flow worksheet, review this section. You probably have some form of laboratory flow system already established. Some of these recommendations may assist you in making it more effective.

- When requesting your due date, make sure that you have adequate time to review the laboratory work before the actual patient appointment.
- Clearly outline borders and margins if you pour your own impressions and trim dies.
- Require your staff to confirm all laboratory case arrivals.
- Clearly write your work orders, leaving nothing for interpretation.

- Package each case separately with its own work order, and label each cast.
- Develop a master log for all laboratory cases and review it daily.
- Use a duplicate laboratory authorization file and conduct a daily review to determine the status of each case and to see if any are past due.
- Know the average turnaround time for each type of laboratory case.
- Review on a monthly basis the number of times patients had to be rescheduled because a case was not completed on time.

BOOKKEEPING/ACCOUNTING RECOMMENDATIONS

If you scored below 112 on the bookkeeping/accounting worksheet, read this section carefully. The proper documentation of your financial transactions is a must. A sufficient number of good commercial systems are available today, making a selection for your specific needs a relatively easy task. Regardless of whether you have a manual system, use a service bureau, or have a computer, the principles of a good bookkeeping/accounting system will be similar.

- Determine if your system has all the essential elements such as:

  A written method of communication with your receptionist (buck slip) that describes what services were performed and what fee is charged for each patient.

  Receipts showing the outstanding balance and the amount paid for that day.

  A ledger or account card for each patient (or family).

  A day sheet that summarizes the charges made, the payments received, and any adjustments and outstanding balances. These totals can be easily summarized and added to other running totals on this sheet.

  A calculation on a daily and weekly basis of all financial transactions for the day.

- Run a tape periodically to match day sheet account balance totals and charges with appropriate ledger cards.
- Complete a bank deposit on a daily basis.
- Run a tape frequently to check bank deposit totals against day sheet totals.
- Use numbered buck slips or transaction slips to ensure that entries are made for all transactions.
- Sign all checks for salaries.
- Use all reconciliation areas on your day sheet to aid you in determining if daily postings are correct.
- Select a day sheet that can break down practice productivity for you. (Applies only to the manual system.)
- Retain copies of transaction slips for use by your accountant to audit data.

PRACTICE BUILDING RECOMMENDATIONS

Scoring below 194 on the practice building worksheet should indicate that you may need to spend more time learning about your patients, examining how you spend your time providing services, and discovering how your practice is viewed by your present and former patients. Reviewing the recommendations listed below should give you new ideas on how to market your practice.

- Assess your strengths as a clinician and as a businessperson.
- Determine the positive aspects of your practice.
- Identify any weaknesses in your practice that you feel may cause patients not to return to your practice.
- List those services in which you spend 80% of your time.
- List those services that provide you with 80% of your revenues.
- Compare those services in which you spend the greatest amount of your effort with those services that generate the most revenue.
- Reduce your level of effort with those services that bring you the least financial return, unless the service is a "loss leader."
- Increase those services that bring the greatest proportion of revenue.
- Determine which services in your practice are profitable by computing their fixed and valuable costs.
- Reevaluate your fee schedule regularly, using the following criteria:
  Profitability
  Patient's perceptions of whether a fee is fair or too high
- Segment your active patients according to:
  Zip code
  Worker classification (such as professional, cleric, business executive, laborer, or housewife)
  Age
- Analyze your recall patients by zip code and determine the characteristics of those patients who visit you regularly on recall.
- Try to attract new patients who resemble the characteristics of your recall patients.
- Provide incentives such as cash bonuses and additional time off for your staff members who consistently bring new patients to your practice.
- Provide incentives such as reduced fees for patients who consistently refer new patients to you.
- Send thank you letters to all patients, dentists, and physicians who refer new patients.
- Improve your communication with your active patients by using some or all of the following:
  A patient brochure
  A patient newsletter
  Birthday cards and other appropriate greetings
  Personal thank you letters.
  A letter recognizing a patient who has appeared in the newspaper
  Personal welcome letters to new patients.
- Conduct periodic patient surveys of regular and recall patients to see how the practice is functioning.

- Use a treatment plan approach that utilizes some or all of the following aids:
    Study models
    Panorex
    Full series (x-ray films)
    Bitewings
    Slides: before and after treatment
    Intraoral photographs
    Charts, diagrams
- Present your treatment plans in terms easily understood by your patients. Try to involve them as much as possible in your treatment plan discussions.
- Develop monthly reports indicating the percentage of acceptance of your treatment plans.
- Maintain a high visibility in your community by such activities as:
    Church group participation
    Community group participation
    School (PTA) group participation
    News columns in community newspapers
    Public service activities

FINANCIAL MANAGEMENT RECOMMENDATIONS

If your financial management goals have not been met, reviewing these recommendations should prove helpful. Reducing expenses and increasing productivity are usually very challenging. However, if you have the ability to monitor both, you should be able to make a noticeable difference.

- Establish measureable goals for increasing your production for the next 6 and 12 months.
- Develop an operating budget for the next 12 months.
- Use your day sheets (if you have a manual bookkeeping system) to total your productivity.
- Use the various formulas on the financial management worksheets (pp. 50 to 54) to calculate percent changes in production and net income from period to period.
- Determine your hourly production and set a goal to increase it for the next year. Use this formula:

$$\text{Hourly production} = \frac{\text{Your production}}{\text{Number of available hours worked}}$$

EXAMPLE:
$$\frac{150,000}{1,200 \text{ available hours in a year}}$$

$$\text{Hourly production} = \$125/\text{hour}$$

- Monitor your expenses on a monthly or quarterly basis by calculating their relative percentages as a function of total expenses.

EXAMPLE:
$$\frac{\text{Salaries}}{\text{Total expense}} \times 100\%$$

$$= \$15,000/100,000 \times 100\%$$

$$\text{Salary percentage} = 15\%$$

- Prepare monthly reports showing the following information:
  Number of recalls that should be seen
  Actual number of recall appointments
  Number of new patients
- Use accounts receivable report to monitor the success of your collection procedures.
- Use the formulas contained in the financial management worksheet (p. 54) to determine your accounts receivable/collection ratio.

Through accurate monitoring you can begin to take corrective action to improve your present situation. These corrective actions can be related to the recommendations for the various applications discussed in this workbook. In addition, you can look at ways to increase your productivity such as the increased use of auxiliaries and the more efficient use of your facility.

Part two
Establishing a dental practice

If you are a new dentist, owning and managing your own practice may seem an impossible goal. However, if you can properly plan your decision and take advantage of the many resources available to assist you, the goal can be attained. This section of the workbook has been designed to guide you through the necessary steps to establish your own private practice. This section ideally should be completed over the course of 6 to 12 months before you see your first patient. Do not be overwhelmed by the number and detail of the worksheets. If you establish a timetable and budget a certain amount of time weekly to completing them, the tasks can be accomplished easily. Much of the work has already been done through the preparation of a framework and methodology that would have taken you months to develop alone.

It would be worth your time to review all of Part II before attempting to complete it. You need to develop an understanding of the entire set of materials and how they interrelate. Some of the worksheets, for example, appear in more than one section of the book because they relate to more than one decision or task. Also, you may want to begin the planning process at a different point than other dentist's. Recognize, however, that the completion of many worksheets is dependent on having made certain prior decisions discussed on earlier worksheets. For example, you must select what kind of delivery system is to be used and the type of equipment to be purchased (Chapter 15) before completing the loan application package (Chapter 16). You should also recognize that all the worksheets contained in this book can be modified or adapted to suit your personal needs. Most of the worksheets provide space for additional items and information and for brief notes.

After reviewing the entire workbook, your first task should be to complete the planning checklist for opening a dental practice. Your progress will be delayed if you fail to complete the worksheet.

11 Planning a dental practice

As previously discussed, the timely use of the worksheets is perhaps as important as their content. Some worksheets must be completed first because all other decisions will be affected by these initial decisions, and other worksheets can be completed just a few weeks before opening the practice. Also, new dentists who have additional demands, such as completing requirements for graduation from dental school or fulfilling a military or public health service commitment, cannot possibly plan to set aside a few months for no other purpose than to prepare to open their own office.

Therefore the use of this workbook is intended to be an ongoing activity. Chapter 11 should probably be completed 9 to 12 months before you see your first patients. Fig. 6 depicts the major decisions and tasks that must be completed before opening your practice. The worksheets that relate to each of these decisions and tasks are also listed in Fig. 15. Although there will be variations, most users should attempt to complete these decisions and tasks in the order presented.

Your first task is to complete the planning checklist for opening a dental office. This worksheet is designed to help you organize the sequence of events that leads to opening the practice. Each of the pages includes a list of tasks recommend for completion during the specified month. The first page identifies activities that should be completed 9 to 12 months before opening. Then you will find a page for each subsequent month including the date for opening your practice.

The column of tasks is followed by four additional columns. In the column titled *Worksheet,* you will find the numbers of worksheets and samples or tables that were designed to help you complete each task. The next colum, *Projected date of completion,* forces you to set a deadline for completing the task. Provision is made to revise the date in the next column. (We know that many factors can justifiably cause you to miss the first deadline. However, no more than one extension is recommended.) The last column is for recording the date when the task /or worksheet is completed. Frequently scan this column to remind yourself of the status of each task for the month.

You will notice that many tasks do not require worksheets because they are simply actions that do not require the analytic framework of a worksheet (e.g., make a telephone call or order materials). Consequently, the space under the worksheet column is left blank. The absence of a worksheet for a given task should not prevent you from preparing one of your own design if you believe that your individual situation requires it. Remember, the worksheets are designed to meet the needs of most new dentists, but you may be inclined to go beyond the structure provided by this workbook.

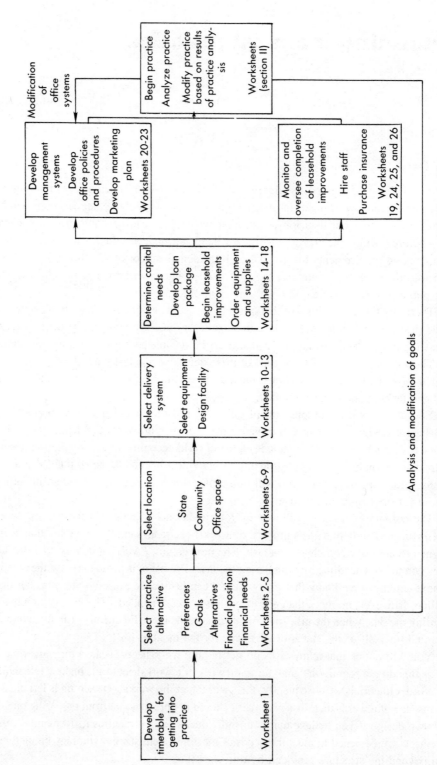

Fig. 6. General schematic of process involved in establishing a new dental practice.

WORKSHEET 1

Planning checklist for opening a dental practice

Time frame and tasks to be completed	Worksheet	Projected date of completion	Revised completion date	Date completed
9 TO 12 MONTHS BEFORE OFFICE OPENING				
1. Develop a philosophy of practice.				
2. Identify your personal goals or preferences for a practice.	Worksheet 2			
3. Prioritize your personal goals or preferences for a practice.	Worksheet 2			
4. Evaluate your personal financial position.	Worksheet 5			
5. Develop a personal budget.	Worksheet 4			
6. Identify potential practice alternatives.	Tables 1 and 2			
7. Evaluate potential practice alternatives in relationship to your personal goals, preferences, and needs.	Worksheet 3			
8. Select preferable practice alternatives.				
9.				
10.				
11.				
12.				

Continued.

WORKSHEET 1—cont'd
Planning checklist for opening a dental practice

Time frame and tasks to be completed	Worksheet	Projected date of completion	Revised completion date	Date completed
8 MONTHS BEFORE OFFICE OPENING				
1. Conduct a preliminary appraisal of practice locations.	Table 3 Worksheets 6 to 9			
2. Determine a desired delivery system.				
3. Develop a list of major equipment needed.	Worksheet 13			
4.				
5.				
6.				
7.				

WORKSHEET 1—cont'd
Planning checklist for opening a dental practice

Time frame and tasks to be completed	Worksheet	Projected date of completion	Revised completion date	Date completed
7 MONTHS BEFORE OFFICE OPENING				
1. Finalize the selection of a state.	Worksheet 6			
2. Conduct a preliminary appraisal of communities.	Worksheet 7			
3. Develop a preliminary loan package.	Tables 5 to 9 Worksheets 14 to 18			
4. Visit lending institutions to determine their general willingness to lend money to new dentists.				
5.				
6.				
7.				
8.				

Continued.

WORKSHEET 1—cont'd

Planning checklist for opening a dental practice

Time frame and tasks to be completed	Worksheet	Projected date of completion	Revised completion date	Date completed
6 MONTHS BEFORE OFFICE OPENING				
1. Select a community in which to practice.	Worksheet 7			
2. Evaluate alternative locations within the community.	Worksheet 8			
3. Contact leasing companies if equipment is to be leased.				
4. Identify potential contractors, architects, interior designers, facility design consultants, and supply houses and solicit information and references on each.				
5. Begin the development of an office policy and procedure manual.	Worksheets 19 to 23			
6. Determine the hours of operation for your practice.				
7. Select an attorney and a certified public accountant.				
8.				
9.				
10.				
11.				

WORKSHEET 1—cont'd
Planning checklist for opening a dental practice

Time frame and tasks to be completed	Worksheet	Projected date of completion	Revised completion date	Date completed
5 MONTHS BEFORE OFFICE OPENING				
1. Select a specific practice location.	Worksheet 8			
2. Obtain, review, negotiate, and sign the lease with the assistance of an attorney.	Worksheet 9			
3. Select a facility design consultant, interior designer, and/or architect.				
4. Obtain facility design and architectural plans.				
5. Solicit bids on equipment and select a dental supply house.	Worksheet 10			
6. Solicit bids on leasehold improvements from contractors, including dates for completion.				
7. Finalize the loan package.	Tables 5 to 9 Worksheets 16 to 18			
8. Apply for a loan.				
9. Continue the development of the office policy and procedures manual.	Worksheets 19 to 23			
10.				
11.				
12.				
13.				

Continued.

WORKSHEET 1—cont'd

Planning checklist for opening a dental practice

Time frame and tasks to be completed	Worksheet	Projected date of completion	Revised completion date	Date completed
4 MONTHS BEFORE OFFICE OPENING				
1. Draw chalk walls and spaces from the design plan, walk through the facility, and modify the plans with the contractor, architect, and/or design consultant.				
2. Sign the contract for leasehold improvements contingent on passing boards and obtaining financing.				
3. Place orders for all major equipment and dental supplies contingent on passing boards and obtaining financing.	Worksheet 13			
4. Review and evaluate telephone systems and answering systems.				
5. Continue the development of the office policy and procedures manual.	Worksheets 19 to 23			
6. Review available bookkeeping systems.	Worksheet 20			
7. Review available patient records.	Worksheet 21			
8. Review available appointment books.	Worksheet 22			
9. Review the state dental practice act and codes of ethics.				
10. Review personnel needs.				
11.				
12.				
13.				
14.				

WORKSHEET 1—cont'd

Planning checklist for opening a dental practice

Time frame and tasks to be completed	Worksheet	Projected date of completion	Revised completion date	Date completed
3 MONTHS BEFORE OFFICE OPENING				
1. Complete board examinations if you are a graduating dentist.				
2. Obtain your license if it is not already obtained.				
3. Obtain final approval of a loan.				
4. Confirm orders for all equipment and general supplies.				
5. Sign the contract for leasehold improvements.				
6. Begin onsite monitoring of contractor's progress on leasehold improvements.				
7. Apply for a narcotics license.				
8. Apply for state, county, city, or township professional or occupational licenses and a business permit if required.				
9. Apply for federal, state, and local tax numbers.				
10. Confirm all equipment and supply orders.				
11. Explore hospital facilities and apply for staff privileges.				
12. Review requirements for unemployment and workmen's compensation insurance and complete necessary forms.				
13. Develop a marketing plan for your practice.	Worksheet 23			
14. Design office stationary and business cards.				
15. Order a bookkeeping system, patient records, an appointment book, stationary, business cards, prescription pads, and other office supplies.				

Continued.

WORKSHEET 1—cont'd
Planning checklist for opening a dental practice

Time frame and tasks to be completed	Worksheet	Projected date of completion	Revised completion date	Date completed
3 MONTHS BEFORE OFFICE OPENING—cont'd				
16. Arrange for a telephone number and a listing in the telephone book.				
17. Make arrangements for the installation of utilities.				
18. Continue the development of the office policy and procedures manual.	Worksheets 19 to 23			
19. Determine the number and the type of personnel to be hired.				
20. Apply for local, state, and national dental society memberships.				
21.				
22.				
23.				
24.				
25.				
26.				

WORKSHEET 1—cont'd
Planning checklist for opening a dental practice

Time frame and tasks to be completed	Worksheet	Projected date of completion	Revised completion date	Date completed
2 MONTHS BEFORE OFFICE OPENING				
1. Monitor the progress on filling equipment and supply orders.				
2. Monitor contractor progress on leasehold improvements.				
3. Finalize and type the office policy and procedures manual.	Worksheets 19 to 23			
4. Finalize your recruitment strategy and place advertisements for personnel.	Worksheet 19			
5. Complete your fee schedule and payment policies.				
6. Explore laboratory options and make arrangements for laboratory work.				
7. Explore pharmacy options and make arrangements for pharmacy services needed.				
8. Explore janitorial service options and make arrangements for services needed.				
9. Finalize the purchase of all professional and business insurance.	Worksheets 24 to 26			
10. Review requirements for unemployment and workman's compensation insurance and submit the necessary forms.				
11. Order the installation of a telephone system.				
12. Design office opening announcements and decide where they will be placed and to whom they will be sent.				
13. Arrange for maintenance service.				
14. Arrange for uniform and linen service.				
15. Join a local credit bureau.				
16. Make credit card arrangements for those that will be accepted.				
17. Complete an application for becoming a participating member of your state Delta plan if a decision has been made to do so.				

Continued.

WORKSHEET 1—cont'd
Planning checklist for opening a dental practice

Time frame and tasks to be completed	Worksheet	Projected date of completion	Revised completion date	Date completed
2 MONTHS BEFORE OFFICE OPENING—cont'd				
18. Decide to which specialists you will refer various patients.				
19.				
20.				
21.				
22.				
23.				
24.				
25.				
26.				

WORKSHEET 1—cont'd
Planning checklist for opening a dental practice

Time frame and tasks to be completed	Worksheet	Projected date of completion	Revised completion date	Date completed
1 MONTH BEFORE OFFICE OPENING				
1. Monitor the contractor's progress on leasehold improvements.				
2. Inventory equipment and supplies.				
3. Hire, orient, and train office personnel.				
4. Complete IRS and other required forms for personnel.				
5. Bond personnel.				
6. Inspect all work done by contractors.				
7. Test all equipment and systems.				
8. Place office opening announcements in selected publications.				
9. Send office opening announcements to selected individuals.				
10. Arrange for the inspection of the office by required city or county officials.				
11.				
12.				
13.				
14.				

Continued.

WORKSHEET 1—cont'd
Planning checklist for opening a dental practice

Time frame and tasks to be completed	Worksheet	Projected date of completion	Revised completion date	Date completed
OFFICE OPENING DATE				
1. Open your office for business.				
2. Monitor all systems.				
3. Analyze all aspects of your practice and make modifications as needed.	All work- sheets in Part I			
4.				
5.				
6.				
7.				
8.				
9.				
10.				

12 Selecting a practice alternative

Starting a practice is no longer as simple as it was in the past. Previously, the only real issue was when the practice would be started: right after graduation or after a few years of military service. Today, however, high interest rates are causing lending institutions to have greater concerns about making loans to dentists who also have big education debts, and the increasing supply of dentists is placing many new graduates at a competitive disadvantage. It is understandable that many new dentists perceive starting a practice as an awesome challenge.

However, the picture is not all bleak. As a recent graduate, you have up-to-date knowledge of modern dentistry and are likely to have a better background than those who graduated 10 or 20 years ago. Also, you probably have had some training in practice management, patient relations, dental care organization, and other nonclinical topics that only entered the dental school curriculum within the last few years. Indeed, today's newcomer to the practice of dentistry has a lot of unprecedented advantages.

The balance between excellent preparation and a harsh practice environment compels caution. This does not mean that starting a practice is impossible, but it does mean that today's dentist must carefully analyze the alternatives and plan accordingly. This chapter is designed to help you complete those tasks.

In this chapter, you are given a framework for matching personal characteristics with options provided by today's practice environment. People choose a career in dentistry for a variety of reasons, and dentistry offers more diverse opportunities than ever before. In the past, starting a practice was easy, but choices were few; most dentists opened a solo or a group fee-for-service practice. The worksheets and accompanying narrative are designed to facilitate the choice and to enhance the prospects for making the correct decision for you.

PERSONAL GOALS AND PREFERENCES

The wisdom of Socrates is relevant for answering questions about practice options: "Know thyself." Know the reason you want to practice dentistry and know the rewards that you hope to gain in the process. Each of today's practice options offers advantages and disadvantages. You will obviously be happier if you choose an option in which the advantages are consistent with your own personal objectives.

Therefore this chapter begins with a worksheet to help you determine the personal attributes that are most important. Use Worksheet 2 to isolate those goals that are of maximum importance to you. Make an effort not to exceed four or five items in the "maximum" category. Expect to take some time to do this, and be sure to involve your spouse if you are married.

Tables 1 and 2 provide information about practice alternatives. The information in these tables is intended to aid you in identifying the three or four alternatives that you might want to evaluate further. You should use your highest priority goals to help you evaluate these practice alternatives on Worksheet 3. Evaluating these alternatives can be accomplished by putting your *ranked* personal goals in the vertical column and up to four practice alternatives in the horizontal row at the top. You can then review the total columns for each alternative to get a rough idea of the relative merits of each. However, the points at the bottom of the columns are only an indicator of the best match. Carefully completing the exercises will help you to find the best match between your personal goals and practice alternatives. The best options will probably be fairly evident before you add up the rating points.

TABLE 1
Potential practice alternatives for new dentist

Veterans administration (VA)
Military
Dental education
Public health service (PHS)
State/city supported clinic
Private practice
  Solo
  1. Begin your own practice from scratch.
  2. Purchase an existing practice.
  3. Sublet space and equipment from another dentist: solo group/time sharing arrangement.

  Associateship/employee
  1. With one other dentist.
  2. With several other dentists (group).
  3. Health maintenance organization.
  4. Retail store clinic.
  5. Satellite office of a dentist.

  Associateship/employee with buy-in or buy-out option
  1. With one other dentist.
  2. With several other dentists (group).
  3. Satellite office.

  Partnership
  1. With established practitioner(s).
  2. With another new practitioner.

  Professional corporation (PC).
  1. Become stockholder of existing professional corporation.
  2. Establish a new PC with an established practitioner.
  3. Establish a new PC with another new practitioner.

Others:

_____

_____

_____

TABLE 2

Potential of various practice alternatives for satisfying commonly stated preferences of dental graduates

Preferences	Military	PHS	VA	Dental education	Private practice			
					Solo	Solo group time sharing	Associateship	Partnership/PC
Independence (being your own boss)	Low	Low	Low	Moderate	High	Moderate	Low	Moderate
Potential financial return	Moderate	Moderate	Moderate	Moderate	High	High	Low	Moderate/High
Flexibility of taking time off	Low	Moderate	Low	Moderate	Moderate	High	Moderate	Moderate
Specific location preference	Low	Low	Low	Moderate	High	Moderate	Moderate	Moderate
Interaction with colleagues	High	High	High	High	Low	Moderate	High	High
Minimize initial financial outlay	High	High	High	High	Low	Moderate	High	High
Minimize financial risks	High	High	High	High	Low	Moderate	High	Low
Desire to do clinical rather than management tasks	High	High	High	Moderate	Low	Low	Moderate	Low
Ability to do research	Moderate	Moderate	Moderate	High	Moderate	Low	Low	Moderate

FINANCIAL EVALUATION

If your chosen option requires you to borrow money or otherwise go into debt to begin, you must evaluate your financial situation and constraints. If you are going to become an employee without financial obligation to the dental practice that hires you, this section will be of less importance to you. However, you may still be wise to budget your personal finances. Some new dentists find themselves in trouble because they handle their personal income imprudently, even when their practices are operating at a profit. Worksheets 4 and 5 are self-explanatory, but you are advised to be conservative and realistic. Completing these worksheets will give you a better understanding of your financial needs and constraints. Ending the first year of practice with an unexpected surplus is much nicer than ending it in debt. Also, loan officers in banks will want to see these sheets when you apply for a loan. This is dicussed more fully in later chapters.

WORKSHEET 2

Potential personal goals or preferences for practice (next 5 years)

Goals or preferences	Importance 1 Minimal	2 Moderate	3 Maximum
Independence (being your own boss)			
Financial return (income)			
Learning from others (interaction with colleagues)			
Flexibility of taking time off			
Time for recreation			
Time for family			
Time for professional development			
Desire to live in a specific area			
Minimize financial risks			
Minimize financial outlay to begin a practice			
Like or dislike of managing a practice			
Potential for growth			
Interaction with other professionals			
Ability to change			
Willingness to relocate periodically			
Ability to utilize expanded duties in practice			
Prestige desired			
Fee for service vs capitation payment			
Type of patients to be treated			
Type of treatment to be delivered (service mix)			
Willingness to adapt to existing clinical and management systems			

WORKSHEET 3

Evaluation of practice alternatives

Personal goals or preferences	Importance 1, Minimal 2, Moderate 3, Maximum	Practice alternative evaluation† 0, = Not compatible with goal achievement; 1, moderately compatible with goal achievement; 2, maximally compatible with goal achievement.							
		Alternative 1		Alternative 2		Alternative 3		Alternative 4	
		R	Total (Imp. × R)	R	Total (Imp. × R)	R	Total (Imp. × R)	R	Total (Imp. × R)
1.									
2.									
3.									
4.									
5.									
6.									
7.									
8.									
9.									
10.									
11.									
12.									
13.									
14.									
			Total ____		Total ____		Total ____		Total ____

WORKSHEET 4
Personal budget protection for first year in practice

Item	Total budgeted per month	Total budgeted per year
1. Housing		
Rent or mortgage payment	$ _____	$ _____
Utilities		
Telephone	_____	_____
Heat and electricity	_____	_____
Water and sewer	_____	_____
Garbage collection	_____	_____
Other	_____	_____
Maintenance	_____	_____
Household insurance and property	_____	_____
Taxes if not included in mortgage	_____	_____
2. Food		
At home	_____	_____
Eating out	_____	_____
3. Existing installment debts		

Type	Balance		
_____	$ _____	_____	_____
_____	_____	_____	_____
_____	_____	_____	_____
_____	_____	_____	_____
_____	_____	_____	_____

Item	Total budgeted per month	Total budgeted per year
4. Insurance premiums		
Life	_____	_____
Health	_____	_____
5. Clothing		
Purchase	_____	_____
Repair, laundry, and dry cleaning	_____	_____
6. Household furnishings, equipment, and help	_____	_____
7. Medical/dental care and drugs	_____	_____

Continued.

WORKSHEET 4—cont'd
Personal budget protection for first year in practice

Item	Total budgeted per month	Total budgeted per year
8. Transportation		
Bus fare or taxis	_____	_____
Gas, oil, and maintenance	_____	_____
Auto insurance and repairs	_____	_____
9. Contributions and gifts	_____	_____
10. Membership dues		
11. Education advancement, newspapers, and other periodicals	_____	_____
12. Entertainment, recreation, and vacations	_____	_____
13. Personal allowances		
Husband (haircut, lunch)	_____	_____
Wife (pocket money)	_____	_____
Child care (school lunch, gifts, dues in clubs, special classes, day care)	_____	_____
14. Savings	_____	_____
15. Federal and state taxes	_____	_____
16. Others: specify		
_____	_____	_____
_____	_____	_____
_____	_____	_____
_____	_____	_____
_____	_____	_____
_____	_____	_____
Grand total living expenses	$ _____	$ _____
Income		
Self		
From practice	$ _____	$ _____
Other	_____	_____
Spouse		
Salary	_____	_____
Other	_____	_____
Total income	$ _____	$ _____

WORKSHEET 5
Personal financial statement

ASSETS

Cash on hand and in banks	$ _____
Savings account in banks	_____
U.S. government bonds	_____
Accounts and notes receivable	_____
Life insurance cash value	_____
Other stocks and bonds	_____
Real estate	_____
Automobile	_____
Dental equipment and instruments	_____
Other personal property (list)	_____
Other assets	_____
Total assets	$ _____

LIABILITIES

Accounts payable	$ _____
Educational loans payable (list)	_____
Notes payable to banks	_____
Notes payable to others	_____
Installment account (auto)	_____
Installment account (other)	_____
Loans on life insurance	_____
Mortgages on real estate	_____
Credit card balances	_____
Unpaid taxes	_____
Other liabilities	_____
Total liabilities	$ _____
Net worth (Total assets − total liabilities)	$ _____

13 Finding a practice location

Choosing a practice location is one of the most important decisions you will make. It is also one of the most difficult and complicated decisions because so many different factors must be considered. This chapter provides worksheets containing detailed lists of the factors that should be considered by a dentist in search of a practice location.

The lists are quite comprehensive but still imperfect. They likely contain some factors that are not relevant to some individuals, and they will surely fail to include one or two that are very important in certain situations. The organization of items in the worksheets reflects a logical sequence that we have found useful when helping dentists choose practice locations, but the progression of concerns will also need to be modified to meet your special needs. In other words, you may want to modify the recommended framework to meet your own aspirations and priorities, but you should benefit from paying careful attention to all items on the lists even though reorganization may be useful. You are encouraged to add, subtract, "cut and paste," and otherwise modify the worksheets to develop a personalized approach for choosing a practice location. However, the workbook's existing format should be quite adequate for most dentists. In either case, you must be prepared to compromise when comparing possible locations on the basis of any criteria. The final choice will hardly ever be the most desirable location based on every single criterion; for example, one site will be the most desirable place to live but another will offer the best income potential. The perfect location is exceedingly rare, so you must look for the best overall place in which to practice and to live. The compromises will be personal and subjective; use of the workbook should help identify potential prospects, but it will not ensure the discovery of a perfect location. Also, be on the lookout for a "diamond in the rough." You may uncover unexpected opportunities and new experiences in the process of searching for a place to practice. An open mind and a willingness to gamble intelligently may pay off. Maintain objectivity, but not to such an extreme that it prevents you from following a good hunch; also, do not undertake the search so seriously that you overlook adventure and opportunity.

HOW TO EVALUATE AND COMPARE PROSPECTIVE PRACTICE LOCATIONS

Worksheets 6 through 8 are designed to assist you with a structured analysis of prospective practice locations. They provide a framework for gathering useful information, and they organize relevant information in a way that permits direct comparison of three potential locations on any given criterion. (To compare more than three locations, use extra paper to add columns for each additional location.)

TABLE 3
Sources of information concerning alternative practice locations

1. American Dental Association, Bureau of Economic Research and Statistics
2. State dental association
3. Local component dental society
4. Dental school(s) serving the area
5. U.S. Department of Commerce, Bureau of the Census, Data Users Service
6. U.S. Small Business Administration
7. State and local government planning offices
8. State and local health departments
9. State and local revenue departments
10. State municipal league
11. Dental supply houses
12. Bankers
13. School district administrators and teachers
14. Clergy
15. Real estate agents
16. Chamber of Commerce
17. Contractors
18. Employment agencies
19. Local dentists
20. Other health professionals (physicians, pharmacists, hospital administrators, etc.)
21. General populace of the community
22. Yellow pages
23. Newspaper classified ads
24. State board of dental examiners
25. County or local zoning department

The left column of each worksheet lists the important considerations. Blank areas allow the addition of uncommon individual criteria, and irrelevant entries can simply be ignored or crossed out. The second column of the worksheets gives numbers that identify likely sources of the appropriate information listed in Table 3. The three columns on the right of each worksheet provide space for recording numbers and comments related to each criterion and location. The small box in the lower right-hand corner of each data entry area allows you to rate each location with respect to the criterion in the left column of the sheet. If the information suggests that the area favorably meets your desires or expectations, a plus (+) should be entered; if the data are unfavorable or otherwise unacceptable, a minus (−) should be entered. The box should be left blank if you have a neutral response to the findings. Multiple entries can be made to express particularly strong or weak factors (e.g., +++ or −−), and special factors can be given automatic weights to reflect their relative importance. For example, you may decide to multiply all quality of life evaluations (+ and −) by two if you consider life-style to be twice as important as any other factor.

On completion of the ratings, tally the weighted plusses and minuses for each potential location and compare locations accordingly. The location with the greatest net number of advantages over disadvantages would be first choice on the basis of the analysis. However, this technique, like any quantitative method for analyzing decisions, does not promise to give the ''right'' answer. It will help focus the choice in some very useful ways, but the final choice is necessarily subjective. The worksheet is like any tool; the outcome depends ultimately on the skill and judgment of the person who uses it.

SOURCES OF INFORMATION

Information concerning practice locations can be obtained from many sources. Because these sources often have differing opinions concerning any given factor, the dentist in search of a location will often be wise to get several observations on a particular factor and to make final judgments (+ or −) on the basis of the overall information. Therefore if time permits, you may want to obtain information from all potential sources for each criterion. These sources of information are presented in Table 3 and identified by numbers that also appear in the second column of the worksheets.

CHOICE OF STATE

Independent of most personal and family considerations, states can be evaluated on the basis of several significant factors. Gathering and evaluating information concerning the factors identified on Worksheet 6 will help you select states with suitable legal and professional environments.

CHOICE OF COMMUNITY

After acceptable states have been identified, the search for acceptable communities (towns or cities) can be commenced. Worksheet 7 identifiies important considerations relating to:

Demography
Economy
Quality of life
Dental environment and competition

WORKSHEET 6
Evaluation of potential states in which to practice

Criteria for comparison	Sources of information	State 1	State 2	State 3
1. Legality of delegation (the extent of allowable use of auxiliaries for expanded functions)	2 24			
2. Legality of denturism	2 24			
3. Mandatory requirement for continuing education	2 3 24			
4. Access to dental school	4			
5. Extent and quality of government dental care programs	2 3 8			
6. Income tax	9			
7. Other				
8. Other				

WORKSHEET 7

Evaluation of various communities in which to practice

Criteria for comparison	Sources of information	Community 1	Community 2	Community 3
DEMOGRAPHY				
1. Current population	1 5 7			
2. Rate of population growth	5 7 10			
3. Per capita income	5 7 9			
4. Median income	5 7 9			
5. Median age	5 7 9			
6. Minority population	5 7 9			

WORKSHEET 7—cont'd
Evaluation of various communities in which to practice

Criteria for comparison	Sources of information	Community 1	Community 2	Community 3

7. Transportation
   Highway system
   Access to air travel
   Public transportation
   Other
	16
	19			

8. Other				
9. Other				
10. Other				
11. Other				

Continued.

WORKSHEET 7—cont'd
Evaluation of various communities in which to practice

Criteria for comparison	Sources of information	Community 1	Community 2	Community 3
ECONOMY				
1. Per capita volume of retail sales	7 9 16			
2. Unemployment rate	7 9			
3. Per capita bank deposits	6 7 9			
4. Availability of bank credit	12			
5. Sales tax	9 16			
6. Property tax	9			
7. Housing market Buyer's or seller's market Housing starts Rental vacancy rate	12 15 17			

WORKSHEET 7—cont'd

Evaluation of various communities in which to practice

Criteria for comparison	Sources of information	Community 1	Community 2	Community 3
8. New business starts sales	12 16			
9. Bankruptcy rate	6 12			
10. Other				
11. Other				
12. Other				
13. Other				

Continued.

WORKSHEET 7—cont'd

Evaluation of various communities in which to practice

Criteria for comparison	Sources of information	Community 1	Community 2	Community 3
QUALITY OF LIFE				
1. Environment 　Population density 　Air quality 　Water quality and availability 　Crime rates	14 19 21			
2. Recreation 　Parks 　Availability of favorite participative sports 　Availability of spectator sports	16 19 21			
3. Church	14 16			

WORKSHEET 7—cont'd

Evaluation of various communities in which to practice

Criteria for comparison	Sources of information	Community 1	Community 2	Community 3
4. Culture	13			
Newspapers	14			
Television (including cable)	16			
Theater	19			
Music	20			
Libraries				
Social clubs				
Restaurants				
Museums				
5. Shopping	16			
Local	19			
Closest major city	21			

Continued.

WORKSHEET 7—cont'd

Evaluation of various communities in which to practice

Criteria for comparison	Sources of information	Community 1	Community 2	Community 3
QUALITY OF LIFE—cont'd				

6. Schools
    Public/private primary
      and secondary
    Colleges and universities
    Financial condition of
      relevant schools
    Accreditation
	13
	14
	21			

7. Opportunities for spouse
    Employment
    Social contacts
	16
	18
	21			

8. Health care
    Availability of
      physicians
    Emergency care
    Hospitals and/or clinics
    Pharmacies
	19
	20
	21			

WORKSHEET 7—cont'd

Evaluation of various communities in which to practice

Criteria for comparison	Sources of information	Community 1	Community 2	Community 3

9. Civic pride
  Appearance of
    community
  Service organizations
  Expected community
    role of professionals
	14
	16
	21			

10. Other				
11. Other				
12. Other				
13. Other				

Continued.

WORKSHEET 7—cont'd

Evaluation of various communities in which to practice

Criteria for comparison	Sources of information	Community 1	Community 2	Community 3
DENTAL ENVIRONMENT AND COMPETITION				

1. Availability of services
    Number of general
        dentists per capita
    Dental specialists
        per capita
	1
	8
	11
	19
	22			

2. Practice characteristics
    of potential competitors
    Age
    Community reputation
    Health
    Office hours
    Apparent busyness
    Average waiting time
        for appointment
    Recent financial history
	1
	8
	11
	19
	22			

WORKSHEET 7—cont'd

Evaluation of various communities in which to practice

Criteria for comparison	Sources of information	Community 1	Community 2	Community 3

3. Dental insurance
  Percent of population
    with prepayment
    coverage
  Extent of coverage of
    prepayment plans
	2
	3
	11
	19			

4. Availability of support
  Supply house(s)
  Dental laboratory
  Potential referral
    network
  Type of specialists
	11
	19			

5. Community fluoridation	3 8			

WORKSHEET 7—cont'd

Evaluation of various communities in which to practice

Criteria for comparison	Sources of information	Community 1	Community 2	Community 3
DENTAL ENVIRONMENT AND COMPETITION—cont'd				

6. Availability of office staff
  Pool of trained assistants
  Pool of workers suitable
    for training
	16
	18
	19
	23			

7. Community attitude
  toward dentistry
    Dental ''IQ''
    Perceived need for addi-
      tional dental service
    Willingness to pay
	19
	20
	21			

8. Availability of financing	11 12			

WORKSHEET 7—cont'd

Evaluation of various communities in which to practice

Criteria for comparison	Sources of information	Community 1	Community 2	Community 3
9. Availability and costs of office space	15 16 19 20			
10. Zoning	25			
11. Other				
12. Other				

14 Selecting office space

After you have found a state and city that best meet the complex blend of your professional and personal objectives, you must choose an actual office location within the city. The attention that must be given to locating the office will correspond directly to the area's population. In general, the amount of time spent for selecting the office location is dependent on the size of the city.

Sections of this chapter identify the basic considerations of office location that should be addressed in all instances. Even in a small town, a new dentist should consider each item on the list to make sure that important points are not overlooked. Larger cities offer more locational choices (and demand more time for careful analysis of alternatives), but the basic considerations of choosing a location are essentially the same in any community.

Designing the office is an important corollary to choosing its location. In the best circumstances you will be able to find appropriate space in the desired part of town, but this is not always the case. Sometimes a compromise will be necessary between the best address and the best space, and you will have to decide which factor should prevail. However, most space can be remodeled, and the compromise becomes a matter of cost and affordability. At the other extreme, you may find an existing dental practice in the desired part of town. Completing the workbook is still worthwhile because it will focus on important considerations that may have been overlooked at first.

The processes of finding a location and designing an office are likely to involve leases, equipment selection, planning, and other important steps that are also covered in this chapter. All elements of preparing to see the first patients are likely to occur simultaneously, so the order of this chapter is somewhat arbitrary. You are encouraged to review the entire chapter before becoming deeply involved in setting up the office. Entries on the worksheet can then be made as the specific considerations are encountered.

CHOOSING AN OFFICE LOCATION

People in commercial real estate have a saying, "Success in business depends on only three things: location, location, and location." This may be a bit of an overstatement, but it is not far from the truth that people will not beat a path to your door if they have to go to very much trouble to find you. Therefore choose a location that can be described and understood with relative simplicity.

Keep this basic idea in mind as you describe and compare alternate locations on the basis of the criteria listed on Worksheet 8. As on the previous worksheets, use the appropriate space on the worksheet to describe the potential location in terms of each consideration, and then use your own judgment to assign pluses and minuses for purposes of comparison.

Be sure to look at each criterion from the perspective of the patients you want to attract. Your preferences were most important in narrowing the choice of cities, but now that you have chosen where to live, let your patients' preferences weigh heavily in the choice of the location within that city. Look at location primarily from the patient's point of view.

EXECUTING A LEASE

Verbal tradition states that leases are executed. You should be careful to ensure that the lease does not do the same to you. Leases must be taken very seriously because unexpected terms in a lease frequently cause some of the most serious problems for tenants, including dentists. This section presents a checklist of considerations for evaluating and comparing leases.

A few specific comments should be considered as each lease is examined. First, the lease should be in writing. A verbal agreement with a landlord is virtually a guarantee for subsequent disaster. Second, the lease should be comprehensible to you before you sign it. If it is too complicated or is filled with lawyers' or realtors' jargon, have the offending sections redrafted in plain English. If you do not understand the lease when you sign it, you can be almost certain that all the incomprehensible provisions are there for the benefit of the landlord in case you are ever required to go to court. Third, the original lease provided by the property owner is not always a "take it or leave it" offer. You should consider making written counterproposals to seek certain terms that are more agreeable to you (such as a lower escalator clause or a greater sum for tenant's finish allowance). Unless the demand for rental space is very strong, you probably have opportunities to influence some of the terms in the contract. If the owner of the property refuses to make any changes in a highly disadvantageous or complicated contract, you should look elsewhere for your office space. Attracting patients to another location is usually much easier than getting out of a bad lease.

Having a lawyer review and help negotiate your lease is mandatory. Also, any rewriting or amendments to the lease can usually be best accomplished by an attorney. Choose one who has experience with leases for commercial space. Do not rely on a real estate agent for unbiased help; in most instances, real estate or leasing agents are representatives of the landlord. Remember, they receive their commissions from the owner, not from the tenant.

Worksheet 9 is intended to assist you in two ways. First, it is a checklist of issues that should be covered in most cases. You should carefully evaluate each lease to see how each issue is addressed. If an issue is omitted, you must decide whether its absence is likely to cause you a problem if something goes wrong during the term of the lease. You or your lawyer will often want to propose revisions in such instances. Second, the worksheet enables you to compare two contracts. (You will seldom evaluate more than two leases; if you do, just copy the list on larger paper and add the appropriate number of columns.) Plus and minus signs are not used in this section because they might give the impression that you should sign a lease that has more good points than bad points. If a lease has serious deficiencies that are unacceptable to you, do not sign it. Renegotiate, or take your business elsewhere. Use the worksheets to help you focus on terms that are important in general situations. If you have special concerns that will pertain to your use of the property, be sure to add them to the list.

WORKSHEET 8
Evaluation of specific locations within a community

Criteria for comparison	Location 1	Location 2	Location 3
LOCATION CONSIDERATIONS			
1. Neighborhood Past history and reputation			
Present reputation			
Future expectations (growth potential)			
Other			
2. Transportation accessibility Private automobile			
Bus			
Taxi			
Subway or trolley			

WORKSHEET 8—cont'd
Evaluation of specific locations within a community

Criteria for comparison	Location 1	Location 2	Location 3
3. Parking availability and cost Patient			
Employee			
4. Adjacent businesses Types of clients/patients			
Exposure to "traffic"			
5. Zoning			
6. Other			
7. Other			

Continued.

WORKSHEET 8—cont'd

Evaluation of specific locations within a community

Criteria for comparison	Location 1	Location 2	Location 3
ADEQUACY OF SITE			
1. Space 　　Useable (net square feet)			
Existing condition			
Electrical circuits			
Heating, ventilation, air 　　conditioning			
Plumbing			
Potential for desired 　　improvements			
Possibilities for expansion			
Other			
Other			

WORKSHEET 9
Evaluation of potential leases

Criteria for comparison	Lease 1	Lease 2
1. Rent provisions		
Base price per square foot		
Escalator		
Rental deposit		
Security deposit		
Late charge		
Legal definition of space rented		
2. Term of lease		
Date of possession		
Condition at possession		
Date for commencement of rent		
Option for renewal		

Continued.

WORKSHEET 9—cont'd
Evaluation of potential leases

Criteria for comparison	Lease 1	Lease 2
3. Provision for use of space		
Allowable uses		
Restrictions on use		
Covenants not to compete		
4. Financing contingency		
5. Default options		
Method of notification		
Time allowed to remedy		
Remedies		

WORKSHEET 9—cont'd

Evaluation of potential leases

Criteria for comparison	Lease 1	Lease 2
6. **Escape and vacancy options**		
Method of notification		
Time requirement		
Ownership of improvements		
Condition of premises		
Definition of uninhabitability and condemnation		
Rights in case of uninhabitability and condemnation		
Other		

Continued.

WORKSHEET 9—cont'd
Evaluation of potential leases

Criteria for comparison	Lease 1	Lease 2
7. Assignment of lease		
Tenant's right to sublease		
Tenant's right on owner's sale or default		
Other		
8. Maintenance		
Premises		
Common areas		
Other		

WORKSHEET 9—cont'd

Evaluation of potential leases

Criteria for comparison	Lease 1	Lease 2
9. **Insurance requirements and responsibility**		
General liability and property		
Fire and extended coverage		
Interruption of business		
Other		
10. **Taxes and payment responsibility**		
Real property		
Personal property		
Other		

Continued.

WORKSHEET 9—cont'd
Evaluation of potential leases

Criteria for comparison	Lease 1	Lease 2
11. Improvements		
Requirements for landlord's consent		
Tenant's right to alter premises		
Provisions regarding liens		
Allowance for improvements included in rent		
12. Common areas		
Definition of common areas		
Responsibility for common areas		
Formula for determining common areas		
Tenant's right to verify charges		
Other		

WORKSHEET 9—cont'd
Evaluation of potential leases

Criteria for comparison	Lease 1	Lease 2
13. Utilities		
Landlord's responsibilities		
Tenant's responsibilities		
14. Signs		
Landlord's right of access to premises		
Purchase option		
Settlement of disputes		
Responsibility for costs of litigation		
Other		
Other		

15 Facility design and selection of equipment

Quite possibly the most exciting but frightening aspect of establishing your own practice is designing your facility and selecting the dental equipment you will use. The importance of these activities should be quite obvious. The rent and leasehold improvements of your facility and the equipment are very costly items and have a major impact on patient and provider comfort as well as on the efficiency of your practice. In addition, once design and equipment decisions are made and implemented, you generally must use them for a considerable period of time. The complexity of design and equipment decisions make it impossible to develop worksheets that will ensure that optimal decisions are made. The worksheets in this section, however, are intended to help you evaluate your initial design plans and equipment alternatives and should provide considerable help in making your final decisions concerning facility design and selection of equipment. For a more detailed discussion of these two topics, read *Dental Practice Management: Concepts and Application,* by Larry R. Domer, Thomas L. Snyder, and David W. Heid (St. Louis, 1980, The C.V. Mosby Co.) and *Applied Practice Management: A Strategy for Stress Control,* by Thomas M. Cooper and John A. DiBiaggio (St. Louis, 1979, The C.V. Mosby Co.).

Before designing your office or selecting equipment, you must make one critical decision. This decision relates to the type of care delivery system you want. There are three basic types of delivery systems: (1) over-the-patient systems, (2) side delivery systems, and (3) behind-the-patient systems. Each of these systems has advantages and disadvantages and require specific considerations when designing your facility. Also, if you have decided on the type of delivery system to be used, you have completed the first step in narrowing the type of certain equipment to be evaluated for purchase. You should make a thorough study of these three delivery systems before making your decision. Read as much as possible about them, discuss them with dental supply house representatives and other dentists, and observe and use each of them if possible. This decision should not be made hastily on the showroom floor based on their physical appearance. Function, cost, and required space should be the major criteria used in making this decision.

Once you have decided on the type of delivery system you will use, have selected office space, and have examined floor plans and architectural drawings, you can begin designing your facility and identifying the equipment to be purchased. Unless you have already developed a working relationship with a full service dental supply company, it is at this point that you will need to select one and perhaps need the services of an architect. Worksheet 10 is designed to help you evaluate dental supply houses. After visiting each supply house, complete this worksheet by rating each supply house on each question and jotting down some brief comments about each. Review this worksheet thoroughly before you decide which supply house you will choose for your business. The completion of this worksheet should facilitate making this decision. Remember that there is one item not included on the worksheet that can have some influence on your decision—prices. However, a cooperative, service-oriented supply house is more important when starting a practice than obtaining the lowest prices.

Worksheets 11 and 12 will help you evaluate the preliminary design of your office space. Whether you do the preliminary design yourself or have someone else do it, you should thoroughly evaluate the preliminary design so that you can decide on modifications to be made before it is too late. Worksheet 11 provides a list of suggestions or criteria for each of several areas that you may wish to include in your office. These suggestions can be used to develop a list of the specific features you desire for each area and the second column provides space for you to list those features. Note that not all areas listed are necessary for your office, but analyze each carefully so that you include all areas that you consider important. When developing your list of desired features, consider the cost of your space, your plans for future growth and expansion, and the function and necessity of each area.

After you have identified your list of desired features, you can evaluate your initial design to determine whether the specific areas are acceptable in relationship to your desired features. The extreme right column on Worksheet 11 can be used for comments and recommendations for modification. Use this worksheet and method on all modified design plans until you are satisfied that the design is as optimal as possible. Remember, however, that the perfect design may not be possible given your space and financial constraints.

Worksheet 12 is similar to Worksheet 11 except that it lists flow and functional relationship criteria to be used for evaluating your initial design. This worksheet should be used in the same way that you used Worksheet 11. You are encouraged to use the criteria listed because they have been proven to be relevant for most dental offices. If you have other criteria that are important to you, add them to the list in the appropriate place.

Selecting dental equipment is the focus of Table 4 and Worksheet 13. Table 4 lists the commonly accepted criteria for various types of dental equipment. This information is provided to help you to complete Worksheet 13. The worksheet identifies most of the equipment that you will need to purchase and includes a column in which you can write the desirable features for each type of equipment. It is recommended that you complete as much of this column as possible before you begin to shop for your equipment. The last three columns on this worksheet provide space to compare three alternatives or supply houses in terms of the degree to which each is compatible with your desired features and costs. If you decide to purchase all equipment from a single supply house, use this worksheet to compare the alternative makes and models available from this supply house. Again, remember that compatibility with your desired features is more important than price, at least up to a point. However, you must also keep your total equipment costs at a reasonable level or you may find that lending institutions will not approve your loan request.

TABLE 4
Suggested criteria for selecting dental operatory equipment

PATIENT'S CHAIR

Operable by either the dentist or the assistant; easily accessible controls

Provides complete body, head, and leg support for the patient in a supine position

Power operated; all segments are independently movable

Rotates on its base (at least 30 degrees right or left of center)

Thin back with no protruding devices (maximum of 2 inches when measured 6 inches from the top) that enables the operator and the assistant to position their legs beneath

Minimum height in its lowest position (the maximum height of the seat would be 14 inches from the floor, preferably 11 inches or less)

Arm rests support patient's arms comfortably

Narrow back (maximum of 8 inches when measured 6 inches from the end) is wide enough to support the patient's shoulders at points further than 6 inches from the end

Single-piece back (not a split back)

Foot controls for raising and lowering the chair

Adjustable, articulated headrest

OPERATOR'S STOOL

Broad base for stability with 4 casters within the circumference of the seat

Separate from the dental chair and freely movable

Large, padded seat; contoured or flat according to the operator's preference

Easily adjustable in height (to a low height of at least 14 inches)

Body support with vertical and horizontal adjustments

ASSISTANT'S STOOL

Separate from the dental chair and completely movable

Broad base for stability, with 5 casters outside the circumference of the seat

Large, padded seat

Easily adjustable height (14 to 21 inches)

Body support with vertical and horizontal adjustments (back, side, and abdominal)

Feet support

DYNAMIC INSTRUMENTATION
High-speed contra-angle

Autoclavable

Water-coolant spray for bur or diamond

Torque is adequate to resist stalling at both high and low speeds

Small head to allow good visibility

Chip blower

Quiet

Easily cleaned and maintained

Locking chuck

Turbine is easily replaceable by operator

Built-in fiberoptic light system

TABLE 4—cont'd
Suggested criteria for selecting dental operatory equipment

Low-speed handpiece

Autoclavable
Torque is adequate at lowest speeds to prevent stalling during rubber-cup prophylaxis or pin placement (below 500 rpm)
Torque is adequate at highest speed to trim acrylic (6,000 to 8,000 rpm)
Quiet
Easily cleaned and maintained
Accepts standard contraangles
Easy-to-use reverse
Chuck mechanism is simple to lock and unlock without a key

Air-water syringe

Combined in one element
Lightweight
Well balanced
Easily operable volume for desired air, water, or air and water spray
Angled tip

High-volume evacuation

Fixed unit (not on wheels and drains directly into waste line)
High air velocity and low pressure
Central power supply
Easily cleaned and serviced
Exhaust outside office
Flexible, noncollapsible hose
Automatic, hanger-type on and off controls
Receives disposable or autoclavable tips
Soft-ended tips (to avoid tissue damage)
Receives connectors to Erickson-type evacuators

OPERATING LIGHT SOURCE, EXTRAORAL

Diffused light, not a spotlight
Easily adjusted from either side of chair
1,000 footcandles illumination at mouth orifice

OPERATORY SINKS

Elbow, knee, or foot controls for water flow
Foot-controlled soap dispenser
Correct height to be used while sitting (height of 30 inches from floor)
Splash-register spouts
Easily adjusted temperature controls

CABINETRY

Minimum number required for storage of essential operatory equipment and materials
Readily available to dental assistant
Mobile module for dental assistant
Proper height for sit-down dentistry

Continued.

TABLE 4—cont'd

Suggested criteria for selecting dental operatory equipment

PREPREPARED TRAY

Located on dental assistant's mobile cabinet
Permits steam or dry-heat autoclaving and convenient storage
Minimum number of double-ended instruments and supporting essentials
Large enough to contain instruments for sequentially planned treatment procedures

OPERATOR'S UNIT

Does not occupy space used by operating team
Does not interfere with patient and staff traffic flow
Quickly and easily repaired and maintained
Accommodates solo or four-handed use
Working surface for the operator
Two electric outlets
Support for radiograph viewing box
Tubing for at least two high-speed and one slow-speed handpieces
Single variable-speed foot control for dynamic instruments
Combination air-water syringe
Height adjustment is independent of patient's chair
Automatic handpiece switchover
Controls are easily accessible to operator and assistant
Mechanism to prevent pull back and torque on the operator's hand

ASSISTANT'S UNIT

High-volume evacuation (HVE) and low-volume evacuation system and an air-water
    syringe
Does not interfere with patient and staff traffic flow
Flexible for solo use
Quickly and easily repaired and maintained
Auxiliary HVE connection
Convenient waste receptacle
Large working surface over assistant's legs
Accessible storage space
Adjustable height

WORKSHEET 10

Evaluation of dental supply houses

Rating scale: 1, No; 2, questionable; 3, yes.

Item/criteria	Supply house 1		Supply house 2		Supply house 3	
	Rating	Comments	Rating	Comments	Rating	Comments
PERSONAL TREATMENT						
1. Are they receptive to you?						
2. Are they courteous on the phone?						
3. Will they give you directions and instructions for parking?						
4. Are they willing to meet you in the evening or on a weekend?						
5. Are you introduced to the other personnel of the supply house?						
6. Are they encouraging and enthusiastic about your practice or potential practice?						
7. Will they begin working with you prior to your receiving approval for financing?						
8.						
9.						

Continued.

WORKSHEET 10—cont'd

Evaluation of dental supply houses

Rating scale: *1,* No; *2,* questionable; *3,* yes.

Item/criteria	Supply house 1		Supply house 2		Supply house 3	
	Rating	Comments	Rating	Comments	Rating	Comments
OFFICE PLANNING						
1. Will they help you choose a location?						
2. Will they help you design a facility?						
3. Will they draw plans and mechanical drawings for an office? At what charge?						
4. Will they give you sample plans?						
5. Will they give you "due dates" for completing financing, ordering equipment, etc.?						
6. Will they give you plumbing, electrical, and carpentry specifications?						
7. Will they work with the construction crew to assure proper plumbing, wall reinforcement, etc?						
8. Will they recommend an institution for financing?						
9. Will they finance you?						

10. Do they charge a fee for their services (mechanical drawings, etc.)?

11.

12.

EQUIPMENT AND SUPPLIES

1. Do they have different manufacturers' systems and equipment on the premises for you to examine?

2. Will they help you choose a delivery system?

3. Do they supply you with information pamphlets on the various equipment?

4. Are they receptive to your equipment preferences?

5. Do they have color and texture charts for their equipment?

6. Do they have a master order book?

7. Do they give instruction on care and maintenance of dental equipment?

8.

9.

Continued.

WORKSHEET 10—cont'd

Evaluation of dental supply houses
Rating scale: *1*, No; *2*, questionable; *3*, yes.

Item/criteria	Supply house 1		Supply house 2		Supply house 3	
	Rating	Comments	Rating	Comments	Rating	Comments
MAINTENANCE						
1. Will they help you organize and stock your office?						
2. Will they suggest order quantities?						
3. Do they offer an inventory control system?						
4. Do they offer emergency repair or service?						
5. Do they offer same-day delivery on most items?						
6. Do they offer and will they inform you of specials or discounts on supplies or equipment?						
7. Do they offer service contracts beyond the warranty period?						

BUSINESS OFFICE

1. Will they suggest expansion or growth?

2. Will they evaluate your billing system?

3. Will they train your receptionist in terms of scheduling, fee collection, etc.?

4. Will they set up or explain insurance policies?

5. Will they provide training to you and your staff concerning equipment maintenance, repair, and care?

6.

7.

8.

9.

WORKSHEET 11
Checklist and evaluation of facility design: component areas

Area/general suggestions	Desired size and features
RECEPTION ROOM Estimate seating requirement by multiplying hourly patient flow by $1^1/_2$. This provides the number of potential people requiring seating. Allow 12 to 15 sq ft for each seated individual. Example: 4 patients/hour, $4 \times 1^1/_2 = 6$, 6×15 sq ft $= 90$ sq ft. Reception room should be a minimum of 90 sq ft. Should convey warmth and concern. Warm colors; adequate reading light. Seated patients should be out of traffic flow. Children's area optional.	
BUSINESS OFFICE Allow approximately 75 sq ft per permanent staff member in the business office. Average estimate 75 to 150 sq ft. Must provide visual and verbal contact with reception area. Must provide work space for business machines, appointment book, files, etc. Should have good lighting and nonglare work surfaces.	
OPERATORIES/TREATMENT ROOMS Size depends on the type of delivery system, equipment, and amount of cabinetry desired. Minimal requirement is 75 sq ft of net working space. Floor space for cabinets is additional. 80 to 100 sq ft for the treatment room is a reasonable estimate. Work environment should be identical in each operatory. Standardization of size, shape, major equipment, and support equipment is desired.	
PREVENTION AREA May be a room or an open area. Should provide the patient with a reasonable degree of privacy. Requires a sink, a well-lighted mirror, plaque-control equipment, etc.	
CONSULTATION ROOM (optional) Estimate 70 to 100 sq ft for this area. Provide a stress-reducing atmosphere. Requires a viewbox, small table, A-V materials, etc. This is an optional area since consultations can be done in the treatment area, prevention area, or private office.	

Evaluation of initial plans		Recommended modification
Acceptable	Not acceptable	

Continued.

WORKSHEET 11—cont'd

Checklist and evaluation of facility design: component areas

Area/general suggestions	
PRIVATE OFFICE Estimate 80 to 100 sq ft per dentist. Should provide a place to read and to do paperwork. Should accommodate private files and a professional library. Should seat 2 to 3 in addition to the dentist, if you do not plan on having a consultation room. Identify the function of this area and plan accordingly. Many people end up with a private office that is much larger than needed.	
RESTROOM State and local codes differ as to size and number required. Usually one restroom is provided for staff and one for patients unless a common restroom is available for patients on the same floor and near your office reception area.	
DARKROOM May serve as a film processing area and storage area. Automatic processing equipment necessitates a larger space. Size will vary from 24 to 100 sq ft depending on equipment to be used and storage desired.	
LABORATORY Size varies with anticipated office labwork, employment of a laboratory technician, etc. Estimate 75 to 150 sq ft. Should be located close to operatories. Sound dampening or soundproofing measures should be taken. *Lighting should be color corrected if porcelain work is to be done.*	

Recommended modification

Continued.

WORKSHEET 11—cont'd
Checklist and evaluation of facility design: component areas

Area/general suggestions	Desired size and features
STAFF LOUNGE (optional) Estimate 50 to 120 sq ft. Could provide room for staff meetings, rest area for coffee breaks, and storage for outer clothes. Could contain a kitchenette, with a sink, refrigerator, heating unit, etc. Location adjacent to staff restroom is desirable. Although there are many advantages to having a staff lounge, cost and space constraints should be carefully reviewed before deciding to include one.	
STERILIZATION Because this area is so busy, it should be large enough to minimize congestion. Estimate 80 to 120 sq ft. Should have adequate counter space for sink, autoclave, ultrasonic, and tray storage. Should have a central location to all operatories.	
STORAGE This area provides space for storage of large bulky items and other inventories. Remember, some storage space may be included in the laboratory, staff lounge, darkroom, etc. A central storage area can minimize the amount of fixed cabinetry needed in operatory areas. The size of this area may range from 30 to 70 sq ft, depending on storage capacity of other areas.	
EQUIPMENT ROOM Should provide space for the air compressor, central evacuation pump and tank, and hot water heater. May need to provide for analgesia and oxygen administration devices. This area need not be large but should be accessible for maintenance.	

Evaluation of initial plans		Recommended modification
Acceptable	Not acceptable	

WORKSHEET 12

Checklist and evaluation of facility design: flow and functional relationships

Criteria	Evaluation of initial plan		Recommended modification
	Acceptable	Not acceptable	
RECEPTIONIST AREA/BUSINESS OFFICE			
Location should be adjacent to office entrance.			
Visual and verbal communication should be possible between receptionist area and patient waiting area.			
It is a support area and should be centrally located for easy communication between patients, receptionist, and operating staff.			
Patients entering the facility should have immediate eye contact with the staff member in the business office.			
Patients should "check in" and "check out" at different counters to avoid traffic jams.			

OPERATORIES

Movement should be around the *head* of the chair rather than the foot, if possible.

Separate traffic patterns should be provided for staff and patients:; i.e. staff movements are at the head of the chair; patient movements are at the foot.

There should be an effective and efficient relationship between the operatories and support areas.

The location of the support areas should be based on their relationship with the operatories.

STERILIZATION

Should be centrally located in relation to all operatories.

Should be located adjacent to the business office to permit staff members to assist each other.

Should allow efficient movement of preset trays.

Continued.

WORKSHEET 12—cont'd

Checklist and evaluation of facility design: flow and functional relationships

Criteria	Evaluation of initial plan		Recommended modification
	Acceptable	Not acceptable	
LABORATORY			
Should be located close to the operatories			
Should be located closest to the operatory used most frequently for prosthodontics.			
CENTRAL STORAGE			
Should be located close to the sterilization area and the laboratory.			
X-RAY FACILITIES AND DARKROOM			
Dictated more by a functional relationship than by frequency of use.			
Should be located near the front of the facility in proximity to the "short appointment" operatory.			
Should be located close to the business office and central sterilization area to utilize available personnel.			

PRIVATE OFFICE

Low frequency of use.

Should *not* be placed close to operatories or other working areas.

Should occupy the "least prime" area of the facility.

OTHER

OTHER

WORKSHEET 13
Evaluation and comparison of major equipment options

Item	Desired features
CENTRAL SERVICES	
Compressor	
Air dryer	
Oral evacuation system	
Vacuum pump	
Analgesia system: oxygen nitrous oxide	
Emergency oxygen unit	
Office illumination	
Other	
Other	
X-RAY EQUIPMENT	
Intraoral x-ray control	
Intraoral arm and head	
Panographic unit	
Automatic developer	
Developing tank	
Lead apron	
Quick developer	
Other	
Other	

Alternative #1		Alternative #2		Alternative #3	
Make: _____ Model: _____		Make: _____ Model: _____		Make: _____ Model: _____	
Compatibility with desired features	**Cost**	**Compatibility with desired features**	**Cost**	**Compatibility with desired features**	**Cost**

Continued.

WORKSHEET 13—cont'd
Evaluation and comparison of major equipment options

Item	Desired features
OPERATING ROOMS	
Instrument delivery system	
Operatory cabinetry	
Dental chair	
Dental light	
Operating stool (doctor's)	
Operating stool (assistant's)	
High-speed handpieces	
Low-speed handpieces	
Contra-angles	
Prophy angles	
Amalgamator	
View box	
Ultrasonic prophy plus tips	
Electrosurgery unit	
Pulp tester	
Glass bead sterilizer	
Other	
Other	

Alternative #1		Alternative #2		Alternative #3	
Make: _____ Model: _____		Make: _____ Model: _____		Make: _____ Model: _____	
Compatibility with desired features	Cost	Compatibility with desired features	Cost	Compatibility with desired features	Cost

Continued.

WORKSHEET 13—cont'd
Evaluation and comparison of major equipment options

Item	Desired features
STERILIZATION ALCOVE	
Autoclave	
Ultrasonic cleaner	
Other	
Other	
LABORATORY EQUIPMENT	
Lathe	
Bench engine	
Laboratory handpiece	
Laboratory stool	
Vacuum investor	
Vibrator	
Model trimmer	
Plaster bin	
Plaster trap	
Casting machine	
Burnout oven	
Sinks	
Cabinets	
Articulator	
Vibrator	
Other	
Other	

| Alternative #1 | | Alternative #2 | | Alternative #3 | |
| Make: _____ Model: ____ | | Make: _____ Model: ____ | | Make: _____ Model: ____ | |
Compatibility with desired features	Cost	Compatibility with desired features	Cost	Compatibility with desired features	Cost

Continued.

WORKSHEET 13—cont'd

Evaluation and comparison of major equipment options

Item	Desired features
PATIENT EDUCATION EQUIPMENT	
Audiovisual	
Visual aids	
View box	
Other	
Other	
OFFICE EQUIPMENT, FURNITURE, AND SUPPLIES	
Chairs (private office business office, reception room)	
End tables	
Lamps	
Desk (private, clerical)	
File cabinets	
Typewriter	
Calculator	
Pictures, clocks, plants	
Refrigerator	
Oven	
Coffee brewer	
Fire extinguisher	
Other	
Other	

| Alternative #1 | | Alternative #2 | | Alternative #3 | |
| Make: _____ Model: _____ | | Make: _____ Model: _____ | | Make: _____ Model: _____ | |
Compatibility with desired features	Cost	Compatibility with desired features	Cost	Compatibility with desired features	Cost

16 Developing the loan package

After you have planned your practice and calculated your financial requirements, you will need to borrow some money to get started. Shopping for the loan may at first seem like a rather awesome task but should actually be one of the easier tasks if you have "done your homework". Working with potential lenders will go smoothly if you present an adequate loan package in a proper, professional way.

The worksheets in this chapter will help you develop the package of materials that should normally be presented to a bank as part of your request for a loan. Complete the worksheets carefully because bankers will examine your loan package thoroughly. You gain at least two advantages from the presentation of a complete package of loan materials. First, you will almost always receive a rapid response to your request from the bank. Inadequate materials can delay consideration of loan requests for weeks or even months because the banks will continue to request more information. Second, you greatly enhance the prospects for approval of your request because a first-rate application will help convince the bank that you are the kind of well-organized person who is most likely to succeed in dentistry.

The value of this competitive advantage cannot be underestimated. Some banks are beginning to turn down requests for dental practice start-up loans because they do not believe the dentist making application is a good risk. A lender is looking for evidence that the loan applicant will be successful. A well-prepared loan application that includes complete supporting documents will impress a banker in many important ways.

When you are ready to submit your loan materials, do not be intimidated by members of the financial community. Banks are in business to lend money; and bankers want your business as long as your practice plans are creditworthy. Indeed, even though banks are now generally more cautious about lending money to doctors, bankers still consider physicians and dentists to be among the best credit risks. They want you to succeed, so their comments on your loan application should be accepted as helpful and constructive.

If a lending officer suggests a few changes in your practice plans, consider them carefully. Bankers probably know more about the financial situation of local dentists than any other interested party. They can be helpful to new loan applicants, so listen carefully and appreciatively if they comment on your application. Bankers would like to help you; approach them as allies, not as adversaries.

When you meet with a banker, act professionally. Dress neatly and be on time. Don't try to impress a banker with fancy talk. The decision to lend you money will be based largely on your application materials. You cannot compensate for a poorly prepared application with a charming personality, but you can fail to qualify for a loan if the bankers think you are pompous or offensive, even if your loan application is excellent. Relax, be yourself, and do a careful job of preparing the following worksheets. If you have a complete application and you know it well, your dealings with a bank should go smoothly.

Worksheets 14 through 18 are designed to help you prepare your loan package. The first two weeksheets are intended to aid in determining whether you will lease or buy dental equipment. Once this decision is made, the entire loan package can be developed. The following items are recommended for inclusion in your completed loan package:

Personal budget

Personal financial statement

Projection of practice income and expenses

Resume

Practice plan

Summary of loan request

A sample and worksheets are provided for each of the first three items listed above. A sample of each of the other three items is also provided. After developing, reviewing, and revising the six items in the loan package, it is recommended that you have each typed and make several quality copies of the entire package so that you can leave a complete set with each potential lender.

LEASING VS BUYING EQUIPMENT

Prior to developing the loan package, you must decide whether you are going to lease or buy dental and other equipment. Worksheets 14 and 15 should facilitate the analyses necessary to make this financial decision.

The completion of Worksheet 14 will provide the total tax savings resulting from leasing and buying the same amount of equipment. After you select the type of equipment desired and determine its price (Worksheet 13 in Chapter 15), you can compute the total for savings (Worksheet 14). Sample 1 depicts a fairly realistic analysis using the format provided on Worksheet 14.

Worksheet 15 provides a means of computing the cash outlay required over a 7-year period for leasing and buying the same amount of equipment. Two concepts that are not accounted for in this worksheet, however, are the concepts of present value and opportunity cost. In other words, if one alternative (either leasing or buying) provides a cash savings over the other, this money could possibly be invested and earn money for you. The earlier in the 7-year period that this savings occurs, the better off you would be because the invested funds would earn interest over a period of time. This and other items such as the total amount of funds lenders may be willing to lend you must also be considered when making the lease or buy decision. Sample 2 illustrates a relatively realistic analysis using the format provided on Worksheet 15. Note that the analyses presented on Samples 1 and 2 are provided for illustrative purposes only and should not be used to make *your* lease or buy decision. You must complete the computations in Worksheets 14 and 15 using your own data to make this decision.

SAMPLE 1

Leasing vs. buying $25,000 of dental equipment: sample computation of tax savings

COMPUTATION OF TAX SAVINGS: BUYING @ 18% INTEREST AND MONTHLY PAYMENTS OF $525.45

Year	Depreciation (straight line)	Approximate interest	Total 1 (depreciation + interest)	Tax rate	Total 2 (total 1 × tax rate)	Investment tax credit	Total tax savings (total 2 + investment tax credit)
1*	7,000	4,333	11,333	.40	4,533	2000	6,533
2	3,000	3,960	6,960	.40	2,784		2,784
3	3,000	3,511	6,511	.40	2,604		2,604
4	3,000	2,932	5,932	.40	2,373		2,373
5	3,000	2,186	5,186	.40	2,074		2,074
6	3,000	1,522	4,522	.40	1,809		1,809
7	3,000	693	3,693	.40	1,477		1,477
Total	25,000	19,137	44,137		17,654		19,654

COMPUTATION OF TAX SAVINGS: LEASING @ SPRING 1982 QUOTES FROM LEASING COMPANY

Year	Lease payment	Tax rate	Total 1 (lease payment × tax rate)	Investment tax credit if allowed by leasing company	Total tax savings (total 1 + investment tax credit)
1	7,950	.40	3,180	0	3,180
2	7,950	.40	3,180	0	3,180
3	7,950	.40	3,180	0	3,180
4	7,950	.40	3,180	0	3,180
5	7,950	.40	3,180	0	3,180
6	1,250	.40	500	0	500
7	1,250	.40	500	0	500
Total	42,250		16,900	0	16,900

*Includes additional first-year depreciation.

SAMPLE 2

Leasing vs buying $25,000 of dental equipment: sample comparison of cash outlay

Year	Leasing			Buying			
	Lease payments	Tax savings	Net lease (cash) (lease payment less tax savings)	Loan payments	Tax savings	Net cash (loan payment less tax savings)	Difference
1	7,950	3,180	4,770	6,305	6,533	(228)	4,998
2	7,950	3,180	4,770	6,305	2,784	3,521	1,249
3	7,950	3,180	4,770	6,305	2,604	3,701	1,069
4	7,950	3,180	4,770	6,305	2,373	3,932	838
5	7,950	3,180	4,770	6,305	2,074	4,231	539
6	1,250	500	750	6,305	1,809	4,496	(3,746)
7	1,250	500	750	6,305	1,477	4,828	(4,078)
Total	42,250	16,900	25,350	44,135	19,654	24,481	869

In this example, the net cash outlay (not considering present value) of buying is $869 less than that of leasing.

PERSONAL BUDGET AND FINANCIAL STATEMENT

Even though you should have completed an initial draft of your personal budget and financial statement to aid in determining which practice alternative you were going to select (Worksheets 4 and 5 in Chapter 12), you must review and modify these before applying for a loan. Since these two items must be thoroughly and accurately completed for your loan package, both sample and blank Personal Budget and Financial Statement forms (Samples 3 and 4, Worksheets 16 and 17) are provided again in this chapter of the workbook. As with other samples, these are intended to be fairly realistic but you should not merely use the figures presented in the sample loan package. You should be as realistic and accurate as possible.

SAMPLE 3
Sample personal budget projection for first year in practice

Item		Total budgeted per month	Total budgeted per year
1. Housing			
Rent or mortgage payment		$ 482	$ 5,784
Utilities			
Telephone		30	360
Heat and electricity		110	1,320
Water and sewer		25	300
Garbage collection		8	96
Other		—	—
Maintenance		35	420
Household insurance and property		Included in mortgage	
Taxes if not included in mortgage		—	—
2. Food			
At home		300	3,600
Eating out		75	900
3. Existing installment debts			
Type	**Balance**		
Auto loan $	2,200	126	1,512
Visa	1,200	72	864
Sears	600	50	600
Educational loans	26,000	—	—

Continued.

SAMPLE 3—cont'd

Sample personal budget projection for first year in practice

Item	Total budgeted per month	Total budgeted per year
4. Insurance premiums		
Life	30	360
Health	42	504
5. Clothing		
Purchase	50	600
Repair, laundry, and dry cleaning	15	180
6. Household furnishings, equipment, and help	50	600
7. Medical/dental care and drugs	20	240
8. Transportation		
Bus fare, taxis		
Gas, oil, and maintenance	45	540
Auto insurance and repairs	30	360
9. Contributions and gifts	30	360
10. Membership dues	—	—
11. Education, advancement, newspapers, and other periodicals	15	180
12. Entertainment, recreation, and vacations	175	900
13. Personal allowances		
Husband (haircut, lunch)	40	480
Wife (pocket money, etc.)	40	480
Child care (school lunch, gifts, dues in clubs, special classes, day care, etc.)	125	1,500
14. Savings	100	1,200
15. Federal and state taxes	400	4,800

SAMPLE 3—cont'd

Sample personal budget projection for first year in practice

Item	Total budgeted per month	Total budgeted per year
16. Others: specify		
_____	____	____
_____	____	____
_____	____	____
_____	____	____
_____	____	____
_____	____	____
_____	____	____
Grand total living expense	$ 2,420	$ 29,040
Income		
Self		
From practice	$ 1,000	$ 12,000
Other	____	____
Spouse		
Salary	1,650	19,800
Other	____	____
Total income	$ 2,650	$ 31,800

SAMPLE 4
Sample personal financial statement

ASSETS

Cash on hand and in banks	$ 800
Savings account in banks	1,400
U.S. government bonds	
Accounts and notes receivable	
Life insurance cash value	
Other stocks and bonds	
Real estate	78,000
Automobile (see Attachment A)	4,000
Dental equipment and instruments (see Attachment A)	1,790
Other personal property (see Attachment A)	4,800
Other assets: retirement (spouse)	7,200
Total assets	$ 97,990

LIABILITIES

Accounts payable	$
Educational loans payable (list)	26,000
Notes payable to banks	
Notes payable to others	
Installment account (auto)	2,200
Installment account (other)	1,800
Loans on life insurance	1,200
Mortgages on real estate	49,000
Credit card balances	600
Unpaid taxes	
Other liabilities	
Total liabilities	$ 80,600
Net worth (Total assets − total liabilities)	$ 17,390

ATTACHMENT A
Itemization of assets

AUTOMOBILES

1980 Dodge Colt	$ 3,400
1975 Ford	600
Total	$ 4,000

DENTAL EQUIPMENT AND INSTRUMENTS

Laboratory equipment (articulator, safety glasses)	$ 70
Instruments and accessories (hand instruments, rubber dam accessories, mirrors, matrix retainers, etc.)	600
Small equipment (contra-angles, handpieces)	800
Dental supplies (burs, files, bunsen burner, die kit, flask press, bowls)	200
Total	$ 1,790

PERSONAL PROPERTY

Household furniture	$ 3,100
Stereo (purchased 1981)	300
RCA color TV (purchased 1980)	300
Appliances (washer, dryer, freezer)	500
Sporting equipment (skis, ski boots, golf clubs)	600
Total	$ 4,800

PROJECTING REVENUES AND EXPENSES

You will need to develop realistic projections of revenues and expenses for several reasons. The immediate reason will be to comply with the information requirements of banks and other lenders, because those members of the financial community no longer assume that a new dentist is certain to be successful. They want to see believable evidence that your new practice will generate enough cash to meet the payment schedule for loans and equipment leases. Indeed, lenders will often vary the payment schedule to fit the cash projections; for example, they might require quarterly payments of interest only for the first year of the loan if they believe that the long-range prospects for the practice are good.

The second reason for estimating cash flow is simply good management. A careful projection of revenues and expenses will provide monthly guideposts for measuring the success of the practice. Consistent and sizeable deviations from the monthly estimates indicate that something needs to be examined carefully. A monthly comparison of estimates with actual performance will allow rapid identification of problems that might go unnoticed for a long time in the absence of a financial plan. Timely response can save many headaches and a lot of money and make the practice of dentistry more rewarding and fun. So, do not look at cash flow analysis as a necessary evil that exists only because you need to borrow money. The time spent on initial analysis will more than pay for itself in the first year, because it will simplify practice management at a time when you need to devote most of your energy to dentistry.

Worksheet 18 is designed to help you project your cash flow for the first year of practice. Most of the items are self-explanatory, but a few items require some detail. Before you begin to estimate your cash flow, read the following explanations and study Sample 5. The numbers in parentheses refer to the number of the item in the left-hand column of the worksheet.

The *number of patient visits* (1) varies with the type of practice you are entering. If you are entering an established practice as either an associate or a purchaser from a retiring dentist, the previous records of the practice can be used to estimate patient visits. For an associate, the minimum number for the first month should be at least six to eight patients per day, and in a solo practice where the former owner will be referring patients, the first month's projection should be at least two to six patients per day. When you are starting a new practice or entering a time-sharing arrangement in which the owner has not agreed to refer patients, the initial estimates will be lower, especially if you do not have your professional listing in the telephone book when beginning your practice. In these situations, a first month's projection of between ten and thirty patient visits is usually realistic.

The second and third months should exceed the previous month, but major increases in patient visits usually occur only after telephone listings appear in the telephone book and existing patients begin referring additional patients, usually between the fourth and sixth months of practice. (Advertising now provides opportunities to accelerate practice growth; see *Personalized guide to marketing strategy,* Volume 4 in this series. By the twelfth month of practice, even a first-year practice could expect to have from 120 to 200 patient visits per month. Established practices usually have 250 to 300 patient visits per month, and some very successful practices have considerably more than this.

The *average fee per patient visit* (2) for the first few months of operation of a new practice normally will be lower than for an established practice because of the disproportionate percentage of new patient examinations, emergencies, and limited restorative visits. An average of the fees charged for new patient examinations, x-ray examination and cleaning visits, emergency visits, and a visit for two moderate restorations is generally appropriate for use during the first 3 months of practice. An example of this procedure follows:

1. New patient visit

   Examination .... $ __20__

   X-ray films .... $ __15__

   Cleaning .... $ __22__

   Subtotal for visit .... $ __57__

2. Emergency visit .... $ __15__

3. Restorative visit

   One amalgam restoration .... $ __33__

   Total .... $ __105__

   Sum of subtotals ÷ 3 = Average fee per visit .... $ __35__

Beginning in month 3 or 4, you can start to use an average fee that is more representative of the full range of care that you expect to provide in your practice. (Considering that a reasonable average gross income for an established solo practitioner in 1982 is approximately $12,000 per month for 250 patient visits per month, an average fee per patient visit of $48 is a good reference point.)

Total billing (3) is determined by multiplying the number of patient visits by the average fee per patient visit. *Total cash available* (4) represents collections. They will be less than total billing unless all fees are collected at the time of each visit (there is no billing or accounts receivable). This figure will vary with collection policies, with the percentage of patients covered by insurance plans that require the dentist to provide or pay a discount (such as for participating members of the state delta plan), or with the acceptance of credit cards that have a discount withheld (such as Visa and Mastercard). Also, if you accept assignment of benefits on insurance cases, plan on at least a 3- to 6-week delay in receiving payment from insurance companies. Annual collections should be at least 95% of billings, but recognize that collections often lag substantially during the early months of practice.

Cash paid out (5 to 30) includes all expenses that must be paid on a monthly basis. Those expenses marked with an asterisk can be estimated quite precisely because they are essentially fixed. Other expenses vary with production levels and are more difficult to project. When projecting these variable expenses, remember that several will be low in the first few months because of consumables purchased for beginning inventory when the practice is established. In many practices, commercial laboratory charges represent between 10% and 12% of gross revenue. This figure will likely be lower for a beginning practice, however, because of a different mix of services being provided in the early months. If as a new practitioner you do your own laboratory work, laboratory expenses will be considerably less. Recognize, however, that if you plan on doing all your own laboratory work, you will need to purchase considerable equipment and that to do so will likely substantially increase the amount of money requested for a start-up loan. You also should be frugal when projecting expenses for conventions and continuing education. Financial institutions would not look favorably on granting a loan to pay for a $6,000 trip to a continuing education course in Hawaii during your first year of practice. For a more detailed discussion of expense items, see the first section of this workbook.

Depreciation expenses should not be included in this cash flow projection. Even though they will be used on an income statement and tax return, no cash is paid out for this expense item.

The *dentist's salary* (27) should be kept to a minimum during the first year. Lending institutions recognize that you must pay for certain personal expenses, but they will not provide funds for extravagent personal living during the first year of practice. These institutions usually like to see other sources of income to help cover personal expenses, such as a spouse's income or income from working in another practice or at a dental school 1 or 2 days per week while the practice is not yet busy.

The *loan payment* (28) represents the payment schedule you have arranged or are requesting from the bank. It should be zero for at least the first 3 months of practice since there will generally not be sufficient cash flow to make any payment—not even interest. Many banks will allow up to 6 months with no monthly payments, but they normally expect payments to cover at least a portion of the interest beginning in month 7. If no payments to the lender are made during the first 6 months, the loan balance at the end of the first year will likely exceed the amount originally borrowed, meaning that an even larger loan balance will have to be retired in 6 years rather than the usual 7.

Operating capital necessary (32) represents the amount of money you will need to cover monthly practice and personal expenses. Until row 31 equals row 30, you have a need for working capital. Funds should be requested in the loan to equal the sum of the working capital needed in each month.

The cash surplus (33) will be zero until you reach the month where total cash available (31) exceeds total cash paid out (30). You should recognize, however, that this may occur early because you are not making any loan payments. Plan ahead and set aside money for the month that the loan payments begin rather than viewing a surplus as spendable income. New dentists often have loan payments of $1,000 to $1,500 beginning in month 7, and those who have not planned ahead may have difficulty meeting this obligation. Also, remember that the repayment of some education loans does not begin until some specified period of time following graduation. Plan for this also.

SAMPLE 5

Sample cash flow projection for first year of practice

							Month							Annual $
		1	2	3	4	5	6	7	8	9	10	11	12	
REVENUE														
1. Number of patient visits		20	30	40	50	60	80	100	120	140	160	180	200	1,080
2. Average fee per patient visit		35	35	35	35	45	45	45	45	45	45	45	45	—
3. Total billing		700	1,050	1,400	1,750	2,700	3,600	4,500	5,400	6,300	7,200	8,100	9,000	51,700
4. **Total cash available (collections)**		400	700	1,000	1,600	2,600	3,500	4,400	5,300	6,200	7,100	8,000	8,900	49,700
CASH PAID OUT														
*5. Rent 850 sq ft @ 12 per sq ft		850	850	850	850	850	850	850	850	850	850	850	850	10,200
*6. Utilities (gas and electric)		120	120	120	120	120	120	120	120	120	120	120	120	1,440
*7. Telephone		40	40	40	40	40	40	40	40	40	40	40	40	480
*8. Telephone answering service		Will be using answering machine purchased from start-up loan funds												
*9. Salaries (staff)		800	800	800	850	850	850	850	850	850	850	850	850	10,050
*10. Payroll taxes (FICA, unemployment, workman's compensation)		80	80	80	85	85	85	85	85	85	85	85	85	1,005
*11. Fringe benefits not included in payroll taxes (specify: _____)		10	10	10	10	10	10	10	10	10	10	10	10	120
12. Clinical supplies and drugs		0	0	0	50	50	100	100	150	150	200	200	250	1,250
13. Office supplies		0	0	0	0	0	30	30	30	30	30	30	30	210
14. Postage		10	10	15	15	20	30	35	40	45	50	55	60	385
15. Commercial laboratory		0	200	200	300	300	400	400	600	600	800	800	900	5,500
*16. Janitorial services		Will be doing this myself during first year												
*17. Linen service		40	40	40	40	40	40	40	40	40	40	40	40	480

*Essentially fixed expenses.

Continued.

SAMPLE 5—cont'd
Sample cash flow projection for first year of practice

							Month						
	1	2	3	4	5	6	7	8	9	10	11	12	Annual $
CASH PAID OUT—cont'd													
18. Legal and accounting fees						200						500	700
*19. Equipment lease	Purchasing all equipment												
*20. Insurance	Premiums for entire first year paid from start-up loan												
*21. Books and periodicals	Subscriptions paid from start-up loan												
*22. Dues and memberships	Paid from start-up loan												
23. Conventions and continuing education	Will not attend any during first year of practice												
24. Repairs and maintenance	50	50	50	50	50	50	50	50	50	50	50	50	600
25. Practice promotion	1,000												1,000
26. Estimated taxes	With tax credits and depreciation, no taxes will be owed during first year												
*27. Dentist's salary	1,000	1,000	1,000	1,000	1,000	1,000	1,000	1,000	1,000	1,000	1,000	1,000	12,000
*28. Loan payment	0	0	0	0	0	0	1,000	1,000	1,000	1,000	1,000	1,000	6,000
29. Miscellaneous	100	100	100	100	100	100	150	150	150	150	150	150	1,500
30. **Total cash paid out**	4,100	3,300	3,305	3,510	3,515	3,905	4,760	5,015	5,020	5,275	5,280	5,935	52,920
31. Total cash available (from line 4 above)	400	700	1,000	1,600	2,600	3,500	4,400	5,300	6,200	7,100	8,000	8,900	49,700
32. Operating capital necessary (line 30 less line 31)	3,700	2,600	2,305	1,910	915	405	360	285					12,195
33. **Cash surplus**									1,180	1,825	2,720	2,965	8,975

RESUMÉ, PRACTICE PLAN, AND SUMMARY OF LOAN REQUEST

The final three items in your loan package are your resumé, practice plan, and a summary of your loan request. A sample of each of these documents is presented on the following pages.

The resumé (Sample 6) provides general information to the loan officer or committee. A well-developed practice plan (Sample 7) demonstrates that you are well organized, that you have justification for selecting your office location, and that you have a firm grasp of the management of your practice. Finally, the summary of your loan request (Sample 8) provides the lending institution with justification for your total loan request and an idea of the terms you are expecting. Although the terms you request may not be the final terms, stating them should help you determine more quickly if a lending institution is willing to consider terms that are reasonably close to those you desire.

After completing the loan package, you will likely find that your total loan request is between $60,000 and $90,000. The two largest items will most likely be equipment and leasehold improvements. Equipment and furniture costs will probably be between $20,000 and $30,000, and leasehold improvements will range from $15,000 to $30,000. Leasehold improvements can usually be projected on the basis of a dollar amount per square foot. Presently, it is not unusual to spend $25 to $35 per square foot for leasehold improvements. Working capital needed will vary with each individual. The amount needed would be taken from line 32 of the cash flow projection for your first year in practice. Office planning and design costs may also vary depending on the amount of service the dental supply house will provide and how extensively an attorney is used. Architectural and attorney fees could, however, be as much as $3,000 in some instances.

SAMPLE 6
Sample resumé

RICHARD L. GREEN (JUNE, 1982)

Address:	2654 E. Ashland Street Lakewood, Colorado 80011
Telephone:	Home: 394-2267 Work: 750-6825
Birthplace:	Lakewood, Colorado
Birthdate:	March 7, 1956
Marital status:	Wife: Betty Birthdate: January 7, 1957 Children: John Birthdate: September 17, 1981

Education:		
	Wilson High School Lakewood, Colorado	1970-1974
	University of Nebraska Lincoln, Nebraska	1974-1978 B.S.
	University of Colorado School of Dentistry Denver, Colorado	1978-1982 D.D.S.

Employment: All employment has been part-time in the summer or while attending school

City of Lakewood Parks and Recreation Department Position: Lifeguard	1974-1977 (summer)
University of Nebraska Lincoln, Nebraska Position: Dormitory supervisor	1976-1978
University of Colorado School of Dentistry Position: Laboratory coordinator	1978-1980
American Dental Laboratory 6518 Montana Court Lakewood, Colorado Position: Laboratory technician assistant	1980-1982

Character references:

Dr. James King (family dentist)
27 E. Alameda Street
Aurora, Colorado 80015
Telephone: 666-3852

Mrs. Gloria Slekton (previous employer)
American Dental Laboratory
6518 Montana Court
Lakewood, Colorado 80265
Telephone: 475-6320

Dr. William Roth (faculty advisor)
University of Colorado
School of Dentistry
6250 E. Tenth Avenue
Denver, Colorado 80075
Telephone: 675-4122

SAMPLE 7

Sample practice plan

Name:	Richard L. Green, D.D.S.
Type of business:	New general dental practice
Location:	210 North 68th Street Lakewood, Colorado 82011
Hours of operation:	7:00 AM to 4:00 PM Monday and Wednesday 12:00 Noon to 9:00 PM Tuesday and Thursday 8:00 AM to 12:00 Noon Saturday

RATIONALE FOR LOCATION AND HOURS

The location is in the growth path of the metropolitan area. Many new housing developments have been built within 2 or 3 miles of the office location because of the aerospace and electronics firms that have recently opened facilities in the area. No established dentists have offices on North 68th Street, the major thoroughfare between the interstate highway and two new housing developments, but a volume retail store clinic is now opening in the new shopping center that is three blocks away from my proposed location. I believe that my personalized, more traditional practice will appeal to the largely white-collar population that is moving into the nearby developments. My evening and Saturday hours will make my services just as convenient as those of the retail clinic. Also, I own a home within walking distance of the office, and my spouse has been hired to teach at the new middle school. We intend to participate actively in the community.

MARKETING PLAN

Considering the increasing importance of marketing for professional success, the following activities will be carried out to promote and build the practice.
1. Advertisement in the yellow pages of the Metropolitan Denver Telephone Directory and the Lakewood Telephone Directory.
2. System of thanking all patients who refer other individuals to our practice. Mechanisms for identifying those who refer patients are part of our standard new patient interview format and form. Standard letters have been developed.
3. Have made contact with four physicians, two optometrists, and one pharmacist who all indicated that my location and hours would be convenient for their patients or clientele. All indicated a willingness to refer patients.
4. Direct mail announcement of practice and practice hours to be sent to all residents within 3 miles of the practice during the first month of practice. Estimate for total cost of announcement design, printing, and distribution through Northern Direct Mail Company is $1,000.
5. Will be working one-half day per week at the dental clinic at the college. This clinic provides limited care to students and faculty but refers all patients needing complex care. No income will be received for this day, but it should be a good practice builder.
6. Will provide 24-hour emergency care during the first year of practice in an attempt to build practice volume.

MANAGEMENT PLAN

An office manual has already been developed outlining management systems, job descriptions, and major policies and procedures. Practice evaluation systems are already developed to assure timely monitoring of practice and identification of potential problems. Have consulted with Snyder Felmeister & Co. concerning the establishment of management systems and the development of an office manual. I will personally supervise all management activities during the first year. Johnson and Associates, C.P.A., has aided in establishing all financial record systems and advised on proper procedures and records needed for tax purposes.

Continued.

SAMPLE 7—cont'd

Sample practice plan

PERSONNEL

Initially one employee will be hired. This person will be a combination receptionist and chairside assistant. A higher than average salary has been budgeted to improve the likelihood of hiring an experienced person. On adding the second operatory and pending adequate growth, a second employee will be hired so that there will be a full-time chairside assistant and a full-time receptionist. A dental hygienist will not be hired until such time that I cannot handle all recalls, cleanings, and other tasks that could be delegated to a hygienist. When this occurs, a hygienist will be phased into the practice beginning with a 1-day per week trial period.

FEES

Fees have not been established yet, but a preliminary informal survey has been done of fees in this area. Many of these are advertised. Fees will be based on a systematic analysis of the costs associated with providing various services and on the fees of competitors. This practice will not, however, attempt to make fees competitive with the high-volume retail store clinic in this area.

Applicant:	Richard L. Green, D.D.S. Telephone: Home 394-2267
	2654 E. Ashland Street Work 750-6825
	Lakewood, Colorado 80011

Purpose of loan: Loan will provide Dr. Richard Green with funds to plan, develop, and begin a private dental practice at 210 North 68th Street, Lakewood, Colorado. Funds to be used for the purchase of equipment and supplies, leasehold improvements, and working capital for the first 6 months of operation.

Total amount of
loan requested: $72,000

Terms requested: Seven years, no payments for first 6 months, interest only months 7 through 12 with no prepayment penalty.

Interest rate
requested: Floating rate, prime plus 1%

SOURCE AND USE OF FUNDS

	Source of funds		
Use of funds	**Loan**	**Equity**	**Total**
Office planning and design	$ 3,000	$	$ 3,000
Major dental equipment	18,000		18,000
Clinical instruments, supplies and drugs	6,000	1,790	7,790
Office furniture and supplies	3,000		3,000
Leasehold improvements	30,000		30,000
Working capital	12,000		12,000
Total	$72,000	$1,790	$73,790

PROPOSED COLLATERAL AND CONDITIONS

1. Borrower will secure and assign life insurance in the amount of the loan and keep it in force for the duration of the loan.
2. Borrower will secure and assign disability insurance in the amount of the loan and keep it in force for the duration of the loan.
3. Borrower will secure office overhead insurance to cover interest payments on the loan.
4. Borrower will secure hazard insurance on office and contents.
5. Loan to be cosigned by Mr. Erik C. Green, father. Financial statement attached.
6. Second deed of trust on borrower's home.

CREDIT REFERENCES

United Bank of Lakewood
127 E. Holly Street
Lakewood, Colorado 80025
(Auto loans)

Western Mortgage Company
117 18th Street
Denver, Colorado 80017
(Home mortgage)

Sears
1134 W. Mountain Drive
Denver, Colorado 80015
(Credit card No. 1-256-440)

REPAYMENT OPTIONS

After completing your total loan request and identifying the amount of funds needed, you should explore potential repayment options. Table 5 presents general information that relates to four options for repaying a $70,000 practice loan. This figure displays the impact of varying the repayment period and terms. Note that there are substantial differences in the total interest paid in the different options. You must not only consider this issue when evaluating terms but also your ability to make the payments required by the various repayment options. Even though you may be able to save more than $20,000 in interest by paying your loan off in 5 rather than 7 years, you may not be able to make the payments required to do so.

Developing a table similar to Table 5 can be done quite easily. The relevant information can be obtained from your lending institution or can be computed by using loan payment tables or one of the newer financial calculations such as the Texas Instruments Business Analyst II.

Regardless of how you complete this analysis, it is critical that you thoroughly evaluate the impact of various repayment options before selecting one. Also, remember that the lending institution may limit you to only one or two repayment schedules. You should be able to compare these with other repayment options in terms of interest paid and your ability to make the payments. If the repayment schedules offered are not consistent with what you want or can handle, you may want to investigate more lending institutions

TABLE 5

Comparison of repayment options for a $70,000 practice loan

Plan/terms	Interest rate	Approximate monthly payment	Approximate total payment	Principal	Approximate interest paid
5 years Equal payments for 60 months	18%	$1,777	$106,620	$70,000	$36,620
7 years Equal payments for 84 months	18%	$1,471	$123,564	$70,000	$53,564

7 years
No payments first
  12 months
Equal payments
  months 13 through 84
	18%	$1,884	$135,648	$70,000	$65,648

7 years
No payments first
  6 months
First year's interest
  payable in equal
  installments months
  months 7 through 12
Equal payments
  months 13 through 84
	18%	Months 7 through 12,
		  $2,100
		Months 13 through 84,
		  $1,597
			$127,584	$70,000	$57,584

before signing the note. For example, if a lending institution demands that payments on interest and principal begin in the first month of practice, you will undoubtedly want to shop around more.

Preparing a table similar to Table 5 for varying amounts of principal will also show you how much less the interest and payments would be if you were to reduce your loan request by a few thousand dollars. You may be quite surprised at how much less interest and payments would be if you would reduce the principal by as little as $5,000.

CHOOSING A BANK

How to choose a bank is not really a suitable topic for a worksheet, but a few helpful hints should save you some time. First, identify local banks that have experience in lending to physicians and dentists. These banks can usually handle a loan application much more efficiently than one that is unfamiliar with the finances of a doctor's practice. Although banks with such experience are generally preferred, an inexperienced bank is not necessarily to be avoided. If it is the only bank in town or if you have personal contacts there, it may be worth the inconveniences.

You can obtain information about different banks from professionals (lawyers, accountants, architects, and other doctors) in the community where you are planning to establish your practice. A personal reference from an established professional can also be very useful. Bankers appreciate referrals, just as dentists do, and they will act favorably toward good comments made on your behalf by someone whose judgment they respect.

Another suggestion is to approach more than one bank if possible. "Shopping around" is generally worthwhile because banks do differ in terms of interest rates, payment schedules, length of loans, and other aspects of borrowing. For example, one bank may offer 2 points over the prime rate for 7 years, and the bank across the street may want 3 points over prime for 5 years. Contact enough banks to determine the range of options available to you in the community; quit searching when you have a good idea of the differences in loan terms. Once you have obtained this information by telephone, make appointments with loan officers at the banks that seem best able to meet your needs.

All other things being equal, you will often get the best treatment from a bank near your practice location. Banks have some territorial identity and they will often favor businesses in their areas. For example, a local bank may give you a better loan agreement if you promise to do all your personal and professional banking there. Since you will usually want to deposit your practice's receipts at a bank near the office for purposes of safety, you should see if that local bank is willing to give you a "deal" on a practice loan in exchange for all your business.

WORKSHEET 14
Leasing vs buying dental equipment: computation of tax savings

COMPUTATION OF TAX SAVINGS: BUYING

Year	Depreciation	Interest	Total 1 (depreciation + interest)	Tax rate	Total 2 (total 1 × tax rate)	Investment tax credit	Total tax savings (total 2 + investment tax credit)
1*							
2							
3							
4							
5							
6							
7							
Total							

COMPUTATION OF TAX SAVINGS: LEASING

Year	Lease payment	Tax rate	Total 1 (lease payment × tax rate)	Investment tax credit if allowed by leasing company	Total tax savings (total 1 + investment tax credit)
1					
2					
3					
4					
5					
6†					
7†					
Total					

*Additional first-year depreciation should be added in year 1.
†Total lease payments for years 6 and 7 are generally 10% of purchase price or 5× monthly payments.

WORKSHEET 15

Leasing vs buying dental equipment: comparison of cash outlay

Year	Leasing			Buying			
	Lease payments	Tax savings	Net lease (cash) (lease payment less tax savings)	Loan payments	Tax savings	Net cash (loan payment less tax savings)	Difference
1							
2							
3							
4							
5							
6							
7							
Total							

WORKSHEET 16
Personal budget projection for first year in practice

Item	Total budgeted per month	Total budgeted per year
1. Housing		
Rent or mortgage payment	$ _____	$ _____
Utilities		
Telephone	_____	_____
Heat and electricity	_____	_____
Water and sewer	_____	_____
Garbage collection	_____	_____
Other	_____	_____
Maintenance	_____	_____
Household insurance and property	_____	_____
Taxes if not included in mortgage	_____	_____
2. Food		
At home	_____	_____
Eating out	_____	_____
3. Existing installment debts		

Type	Balance		
_____	$ _____	_____	_____
_____	_____	_____	_____
_____	_____	_____	_____
_____	_____	_____	_____
_____	_____	_____	_____

Item	Total budgeted per month	Total budgeted per year
4. Insurance premiums		
Life	_____	_____
Health	_____	_____
5. Clothing		
Purchase	_____	_____
Repair, laundry, and dry cleaning	_____	_____
6. Household furnishings, equipment, and help	_____	_____
7. Medical/dental care, and drugs	_____	_____

WORKSHEET 16—cont'd
Personal budget projection for first year in practice

Item	Total budgeted per month	Total budgeted per year
8. Transportation		
Bus fare, taxis	_____	_____
Gas, oil, and maintenance	_____	_____
Auto insurance and repairs	_____	_____
9. Contributions and gifts	_____	_____
10. Membership dues	_____	_____
11. Education, advancement, newspapers, and other periodicals	_____	_____
12. Entertainment, recreation, and vacations	_____	_____
13. Personal allowances		
Husband (haircut, lunch)	_____	_____
Wife (pocket money)	_____	_____
Child care (school lunch, gifts, dues in clubs, special classes, day care)	_____	_____
14. Savings	_____	_____
15. Federal and state taxes	_____	_____
16. Others: specify		
_____	_____	_____
_____	_____	_____
_____	_____	_____
_____	_____	_____
_____	_____	_____
_____	_____	_____
Grand total living expense	$ _____	$ _____
Income		
Self		
From practice	$ _____	$ _____
Other	_____	_____
Spouse		
Salary	_____	_____
Other	_____	_____
Total income	$ _____	$ _____

WORKSHEET 17
Personal financial statement

ASSETS

Cash on hand and in banks $ _____

Savings accounts in banks   _____

U.S. government bonds   _____

Accounts and notes receivable   _____

Life insurance cash value   _____

Other stocks and bonds   _____

Real estate   _____

Automobile   _____

Dental equipment and instruments   _____

Other personal property (list)   _____

Other assets   _____

Total assets

LIABILITIES

Accounts payable $ _____

Educational loans payable (list)   _____

Notes payable to banks   _____

Notes payable to others   _____

Installment account (auto)   _____

Installment account (other)   _____

Loans on life insurance   _____

Mortgages on real estate   _____

Credit card balances   _____

Unpaid taxes   _____

Other liabilities   _____

Total liabilities $ _____

Net worth (Total assets − total liabilities) $ _____

WORKSHEET 18

Cash flow projection for first year of practice

	Month												Annual $
	1	2	3	4	5	6	7	8	9	10	11	12	
REVENUE													
1. Number of patient visits													
2. Average fee per patient visit													
3. Total billing													
4. **Total cash available (collections)**													
CASH PAID OUT													
* 5. Rent ____ sq ft @ ____ per sq ft													
* 6. Utilities (gas and electric)													
* 7. Telephone													
* 8. Telephone answering service													
* 9. Salaries (staff)													
*10. Payroll taxes (FICA, unemployment, workman's compensation)													
*11. Fringe benefits not included in payroll taxes (specify: ____)													
12. Clinical supplies and drugs													
13. Office supplies													
14. Postage													
15. Commercial laboratory													
*16. Janitorial services													
*17. Linen service													

*Essentially fixed expenses.

Continued.

WORKSHEET 18—cont'd

Cash flow projection for first year of practice

	Month												Annual $
	1	2	3	4	5	6	7	8	9	10	11	12	
CASH PAID OUT—cont'd													
18. Legal and accounting fees													
*19. Equipment lease													
*20. Insurance													
*21. Books and periodicals													
*22. Dues and memberships													
23. Conventions and continuing education													
24. Repairs and maintenance													
25. Practice promotion													
26. Estimated taxes													
*27. Dentist's salary													
*28. Loan payment													
29. Miscellaneous													
30. **Total cash paid out**													
31. Total cash available (from line 4 above)													
32. Operating capital necessary (line 30 less line 31)													
33. **Cash surplus**													

17 Management and operational systems

Finding a location, obtaining financing, and completing your facility make it possible for you to begin the practice of dentistry. It is impossible to begin practice until these things are accomplished. Unfortunately, however, many dentists expend so much time and energy in accomplishing them that they do not devote sufficient thought or effort to planning and designing the systems that will make the practice function efficiently and effectively. As depicted in Worksheet 1, Planning Checklist for Opening a Dental Practice, there are many systems, policies, and procedures that must be developed and in operation prior to opening your practice. The following pages have been designed to aid in the identification and development of important systems, policies, and procedures for your new practice. As with other worksheets and figures presented in this workbook, the ones in this chapter provide a framework for developing practice systems but do not dictate how these systems should be developed.

Individual and location differences will likely cause your systems and policies to differ from those of other dentists. The important thing is that you conscientiously develop the systems, policies, and procedures identified here before you are actively engaged in practice.

The left columns of Worksheets 19 through 23 provide comprehensive lists of items for which policies, procedures, or plans should be developed and questions that should be answered prior to beginning practice. The next column in each worksheet provides space to enter a target date for completing each of the policies, procedures, plans, or decisions. The largest column provides space to write your initial draft of these policies, procedures, or decisions. Items requiring more space than provided should be written on additional pages and inserted in the appropriate section of this workbook. The far right columns provide space to indicate when each policy or procedure has been finalized, typed, and inserted in your office manual or to indicate that other nonpolicy and procedure items have been handled to your satisfaction (e.g., a pegboard system has been selected and ordered).

WORKSHEET 19

Policies and procedures development checklist: personnel system

Item/question	Target date for completion	Brief description of your policy, procedure, or decision	Final draft completed
RECRUITMENT AND SELECTION			
What type of employee will be hired first?			
When do you want this person to start?			
What does this person's job description include?			
How will you advertise for the position? When?			
What will the advertisement include?			

What are the minimum qualifications desired?						
How will you screen applicants?						
Selection of application blank to be used						
Development of telephone screening format						
Development of interviewing protocol (how many, how long, format)						
Reference check policy and procedures						
How will you orient and train your first employee?						

Continued.

WORKSHEET 19—cont'd

Policies and procedures development checklist: personnel system

Item/question	Target date for completion	Brief description of your policy, procedure, or decision	Final draft completed
EMPLOYMENT POLICIES			
Beginning salary			
How raises will be determined and when			
Incentive systems to be used, if any			
Fringe benefits provided: Vacation: How much? When are employees eligible? How must it be scheduled?			
Sick leave: How much? How does it accrue? When can it be used? Can it be carried over into the next year? Will you pay for unused sick leave? If so, how much?			

Insurance						
Retirement						
Uniform allowance						
Participation in continuing education courses						
Dental care for self and family						
Probationary period						
Hours of work and attendance						

Continued.

WORKSHEET 19—cont'd

Policies and procedures development checklist: personnel system

Item/question	Target date for completion	Brief description of your policy, procedure, or decision	Final draft completed
EMPLOYMENT POLICIES—cont'd			
Holidays (paid or not; which ones)			
Leave policy (maternity, jury duty, military, death in family)			
Performance evaluation (how, when, is salary affected?)			
Promotions and advancement			
Personal appearance			

Dress code						
Personal conduct						
Smoking						
Breaks						
Bonding						
Overtime pay						
Uniform code						

Continued.

WORKSHEET 19—cont'd

Policies and procedures development checklist: personnel system

Item/question	Target date for completion	Brief description of your policy, procedure, or decision	Final draft completed
EMPLOYMENT POLICIES—cont'd			
Dismissal			
Severance pay			
Employment of relatives			
Equal employment opportunity			
Staff meetings			
Use of telephone for personal business			

WORKSHEET 20

Policies and procedures development checklist: bookkeeping system

Item/question	Target date for completion	Brief description of your policy, procedure, or decision	Final draft completed
RECEIPTS AND ACCOUNTS RECEIVABLE **Pegboard system**			
Day sheet (should have adjustments column, tear-off bank deposit slip, and easy to understand page proof system)			
Ledger cards and filing system			
Numbered transaction slips			
Filing system for transaction slips			
Receipts			
Procedures for completing these documents (who, how, when?)			

Continued.

WORKSHEET 20—cont'd

Policies and procedures development checklist: bookkeeping system

Item/question	Target date for completion	Brief description of your policy, procedure, or decision	Final draft completed
RECEIPTS AND ACCOUNTS RECEIVABLE—cont'd			
Collections			
Payment policy (cash, credit cards, bill, combination)			
Method of informing patients of your policy (how, who does it?)			
Are you going to provide a receipt for each visit stating balance due and self-addressed envelope to encourage prompt payment?			
Billing			
Method of billing (photocopy ledger card, prepare statements as you go, statements prepared at end of month, computer service bureau)			
When you will bill (end of month, middle of month, combination)?			

Extent of itemization on bills

Aging of balance on bills

Follow-up policies and procedures for past due accounts (when does follow-up process begin, what will it be—telephone call, letter, etc.)

Insurance

Will you accept assignments of benefits? (yes, no, sometimes)

Is there a minimum charge per visit that you expect patients to pay at time of treatment, but if visit exceeds this, you will bill insurance company directly?

Do you expect patients to pay for initial and emergency visits and be reimbursed by the insurance company?

Continued.

WORKSHEET 20—cont'd

Policies and procedures development checklist: bookkeeping system

Item/question	Target date for completion	Brief description of your policy, procedure, or decision	Final draft completed
RECEIPTS AND ACCOUNTS RECEIVABLE—cont'd **Insurance—cont'd**			
Method of informing patients of your policy			
Copayment policy (patient pays portion as treatment is rendered vs billing patient after all treatment and after you receive payment from insurance company)			
Method of handling copayment on statements			
Insurance log (type and responsibility for entries)			
Aging of insurance accounts receivable			

Continued.

Follow-up procedures for overdue preauthorization and insurance payments (how, who will do it, when)				
Medicaid policies (will you accept Medicaid and if so, method of follow-up)				
Will you request preauthorization for cases exceeding $200?				
How often will claim forms be submitted to insurance companies (daily, weekly, monthly, or when all treatment for patient is completed)?				
Type of claim form to be used (patients', American Dental Association standardized claim form, super bill)				

WORKSHEET 20—cont'd

Policies and procedures development checklist: bookkeeping system

Item/question	Target date for completion	Brief description of your policy, procedure, or decision	Final draft completed
RECEIPTS AND ACCOUNTS RECEIVABLE—cont'd **Control and protection**			
How often will you sum balances on ledger cards and compare with accounts receivable balance on day sheet?			
How often will you review transaction slips and compare with day sheet entries?			
How often will you review day sheets to check for unusual entries, cross outs, erasures, etc.?			
Mechanisms for protection of financial records (copies, fireproof storage, etc.)			
How often and when will bank deposit slips be compared to day sheet totals?			
Deposit policies (who, when?)			
Petty cash amount, policies, and records			

ACCOUNTS PAYABLE

Check writing system (pegboard, other)						
Expense categories for record-keeping purposes						
Who will write checks?						
When will checks be written?						
Filing system for orders, invoices, bills, etc.						
Payroll records						
Pay periods for employees						

WORKSHEET 21

Policies and procedures development checklist: clinical record system

Item/question	Target date for completion	Brief description of your policy, procedure, or decision	Final draft completed
Patient health questionnaire completed by patients (type, when is it to be completed?)			
Health history form completed for office personnel (type)			
Dental chart (type, notations to be used, treatment plan, progress notes, filing system)			
Consent forms (content, when required)			

Requisitions for laboratory work (type, filing)	Radiographs (type, policy concerning providing patient copies)	Diagnostic casts (labeling, filing, storing)	Intraoral photographs (policy, procedure, consent forms if you intend to use them in public)

WORKSHEET 22

Policies and procedures development checklist: appointment scheduling system

Item/question	Target date for completion	Brief description of your policy, procedure, or decision	Final draft completed
Type of appointment book (style, time units desired)			
Standard notations to be used in appointment book			
Standard information to be written in appointment book for each patient appointment			
New patient appointment (procedure to be done, how long it will take)			

Time estimates for procedures				
Broken appointment policy				
Mechanism for following up on broken and cancelled appointments				
Short-notice call list to fill broken and cancelled appointments				
Method of informing patients of your policy				
Confirmation of appointments (will you, when)				

Continued.

WORKSHEET 22—cont'd

Policies and procedures development checklist: appointment scheduling system

Item/question	Target date for completion	Brief description of your policy, procedure, or decision	Final draft completed
Mechanism for reviewing and posting daily schedule			
Emergency patients			
Double booking			
Overlap scheduling			

Time preferences for scheduling certain types of appointments (pedodontic, case presentations, crown and bridge, etc.)	Other scheduling preferences (not scheduling two endodontic appointments in a row, etc.)	Responsibility for appointment scheduling (who)	Recall system (type, implementation, who will be responsible)	Follow-up system for patients not scheduling recall appointments

WORKSHEET 23

Policies and procedures development checklist: marketing system

Item/question	Target date for completion	Brief description of your policy, procedure, or decision	Final draft completed
Objectives for growth			
Mechanism for determining how patients learned about your practice			
Type of telephone listing			
New practice announcements			

Advertising plans, if any (newsletter, direct mail advertising, mass media advertising)			
Other promotional plans			
Mechanism for thanking people who refer patients to you (method [letters, gifts, telephone calls], after how many referrals, content of message)			
Hours of operation (evenings and weekends may be helpful)			

18 Professional and business insurance

Before seeing your first patient, you must have insurance coverage in effect. In fact the day you sign your lease and begin renovations you should have most insurance coverage in effect. Beginning that day, you expose yourself and your property to certain risks. Although the types and amounts of insurance coverage needed will vary, most new practitioners who have their own office will need coverage in several basic areas.

Worksheets 24 through 26 are designed to help identify the types of coverage you need and want and to compare the costs of obtaining these coverages from alternative companies. The left column of Worksheet 24 lists most types of coverage that you may purchase. The next three columns identify those types of coverage that are required, those that are recommended, and those that are optional. You should not be without those indicated as required. If possible you should also strongly consider purchasing the types of coverage identified as recommended. The optional types of coverage may be purchased but are not necessary in most situations.

Your first task is to complete the far right column of Worksheet 24 by checking those types of coverage you want to purchase. Discussions with insurance agents, review of American Dental Association and state association group plans, and additional reading may be necessary to complete this task.

Worksheet 25 provides a framework for identifying the features you want in each type of coverage. You should identify the features you want before comparing premiums for policies from alternative companies. If you do not, you are likely to find yourself comparing apples to oranges. For example, disability policies may or may not be non-cancelable and guaranteed renewable. Also, policies can be for varying amounts and can have different waiting periods and benefit periods. The definition of disability also varies from one policy to another, and policies may or may not provide benefits for partial disability. Sample 9 illustrates the manner in which you complete Worksheet 25. After you have identified the features you want in each type of coverage desired, you should list questions that you would like to have answered concerning the coverage provided in alternative policies. When you have completed this worksheet, you can give it to one or more insurance agents and tell them to quote you their premiums for the desired coverage and provide answers to your questions. If Worksheet 25 is completed and used in this manner, it should save you considerable time with insurance agents.

If you decide to get premium quotes from more than one insurance agent for the same coverage, you can use Worksheet 26 to compare these quotes and the coverage provided. Make sure you list the variations from the desired features listed on Worksheet 25. Remember, variations in premiums are usually the result of one policy having different features and terms than another. Once you have completed Worksheet 25, you can decide which agent offers coverage closest to what you want for the most reasonable premium. Unfortunately, you will likely find that the same agent does not provide the best coverage for the lowest premium on all coverages desired. You must then decide if you are going to purchase all coverage from a single agent or purchase coverages from several agents. If the premium differences are substantial, you may want to purchase coverages from several agents, but if they are not, you should consider working with only one agent. Remember, you need an insurance advisor to keep you informed of changes in insurance and to help you monitor your coverage in light of changes in your practice and personal situation. Also, when the need arises, you want someone who will help with the prompt and speedy processing of claims so you or your estate can receive insurance benefits. These things are more likely to occur if you have one or two insurance agents rather than many.

SAMPLE 9

Sample features desired in policies to be purchased

Type of policy or coverage	Desired features	Questions to ask
Life insurance	Coverage: $150,000 5-year renewable term Waiver of premium	1. What are conversion options —to whole life only or to other term policies such as decreasing term? 2. What is the difference in premium for annual renewable and ten year renewable policies?

Disability insurance	Coverage: $2,500/month
	Noncancelable,
	   guaranteed renewable
	30-day waiting period
	Sickness benefits to age 65
	Accident benefits for life
	Waiver of premium
	Partial disability coverage
		1. What is definition of:
		  a. Total disability?
		  b. Partial disability?
		2. Partial disability:
		  a. What percent of loss must be incurred to collect?
		  b. How is prior income determined? Length of time partial benefits are provided?
		  c. What does the policy consider as income after you return to your practice?
		  d. Does the policy make adjustments for inflation?

WORKSHEET 24
Checklist of potential insurance policies or coverage

Type of policy or coverage	Required	Recommended	Optional	Selected
Liability insurance				
Professional	X			
Office premise	X			
Medical payments		X		
Public liability	X			
Employer's liability: employees	X			
Personal injury	X			
Automobile				
Owned vehicles	X			
Nonowned vehicles	X			
Rented vehicles	X			
Personal excess coverage (umbrella policy)	X			
Property insurance				
Operating and office equipment and contents	X			
In transit		X		
Office records and money		X		
Patient charts		X		
X-ray films		X		
Accounts receivable		X		
Practice interruption		X		
Extended coverage		X		
Vandalism: building and contents			X	
Sprinkler leakage: building and contents			X	

WORKSHEET 24—cont'd
Checklist of potential insurance policies or coverage

Type of policy or coverage	Required	Recommended	Optional	Selected
Life insurance	X			
Disability insurance		X		
Overhead insurance		X		
Employee dishonesty insurance	X			
Workman's compensation insurance	X			
Group medical insurance		X		
Major medical insurance	X			
Homeowner's insurance	X			

WORKSHEET 25

Features desired in policies to be purchased

Type of policy or coverage	Desired features	Questions to ask

WORKSHEET 26

Comparing costs of alternative insurance policies or coverages

Type of policy or coverage	Policy 1 Company: _____	
	Variations from desired features	Annual premium: ___

Policy 2 Company: _____		Annual premium: _____	Policy 3 Company: _____		Annual premium: _____
Variations from desired features			**Variations from desired features**		

Index